A Compendium of TCM Patterns & Treatments

A Compendium of TCM Patterns & Treatments

Bob Flaws
Daniel Finney

BLUE POPPY PRESS
BOULDER, CO

Published by:

BLUE POPPY PRESS, INC.
1775 LINDEN AVE.
BOULDER, CO 80304

First Edition, January, 1996

ISBN 0-936185-70-8
LC 95-83250

The information in this book is given in good faith. However, the authors
and the publishers cannot be held responsible for any error or omission. Nor can they be
held in any way responsible for treatment given on the basis of information contained in this book.
The publishers make this information available to readers
for scholarly and research purposes only.

The publishers do not advocate nor endorse self-medication by laypersons.
Chinese medicine is a professional medicine. Laypersons interested in availing
themselves of the treatments described in this book should seek out a qualified
professional practitioner of Chinese medicine.

COMP Designation: Original work using a standard translational terminology for
Chinese medical technical terms

Printed at Johnson Printing in Boulder, CO on acid free,
recycled, elementally chlorine-free paper

10 9 8 7 6 5 4 3 2

Preface

As a student in an American school of TCM, when moving from the classroom to the student clinic, it quickly became apparent to me that Western patients seldom fit the exact mold of a single pattern as described in introductory English language textbooks on TCM. Furthermore, Western patients commonly present a myriad of signs and symptoms that can leave the student overwhelmed when trying to discriminate just one or even a two part pattern. Many times when I first started in student clinic, I would use liver depression, qi stagnation and spleen qi vacuity as a security blanket in complex cases instead of really trying to decipher what was truly going on. And at that time I really did not find a single English language book that could guide me in making more complex pattern discriminations.

Happily, after helping Bob Flaws work on this book for several months and also using it in the classroom and student clinic, it has become much easier for me to recognize which patterns and pattern combinations are the most prevalent in Western clinical practice. In addition, this book has helped make complicated cases clearer. For example, it is not uncommon to see liver depression, qi stagnation with depressive heat, spleen qi vacuity, blood vacuity, and blood stasis coupled with damp heat in the lower burner causing or at least accompanying kidney yang vacuity. This complex pattern is not discussed as such in any other English language texts, but does present in Western clinical practice on a regular basis. If one only sees and therefore only treats the elements of liver depression, qi stagnation and spleen qi vacuity, either the patient will only get partially better or will only get better for a short while and then relapse.

Western patients seeking treatment from acupuncturists and practitioners of Traditional Chinese Medicine tend to be what in China are referred to as knotty, difficult to treat patients. The others have either been successfully treated by other practitioners or have gotten better because their condition was self-limiting. We, on the other hand, are typically care providers of last resource, and as Bob is fond of saying, we have to be better Chinese doctors than the typical doctor in China. Therefore, it is our hope that this book will help both students and practitioners to gain greater clarity and accuracy in their in clinical application of TCM pattern discrimination.

The technical terminology used throughout this book for all TCM terms and concepts is based on Nigel Wiseman's *Glossary of Chinese Medical Terms and Acupuncture Points*, Paradigm Publications, Brookline, MA, 1990. In terms of acupuncture nomenclature, we have also used Wiseman's *Glossary* except that we have abbreviated the channel identifications as follows: Lu for Lung, LI for Large Intestine, St for Stomach, Sp for Spleen, Ht for Heart, SI for Small Intestine, Bl for Bladder, Ki for Kidney, Per for Pericardium, TB for Triple Burner, GB for Gallbladder, Liv for Liver, CV for Conception Vessel, and GV for Governing Vessel.

Daniel Finney
Boulder, CO
November 27, 1995

Contents

Introduction
TCM Pattern Discrimination

This book is a compendium of Traditional Chinese Medicine (TCM) pattern discrimination and treatment. By TCM, we mean that style of Chinese medicine that is the dominant style taught at the provincial Chinese medical colleges in the Peoples' Republic of China today. The key defining statement of this style is *bian zheng lun zhi,* the basing of treatment on pattern discrimination. The following couplet is an extension and explanation of this methodology of basing treatment on pattern discrimination:

> *Yi bing, tong zhi;*
> *Tong bing, yi zhi.*

> One disease, different treatments;
> Different diseases, one treatment.

This means that two patients with the same named disease diagnosis may receive entirely different treatments if their TCM pattern discrimination is different, while two patients with different disease diagnoses may receive the same treatment if their TCM pattern discrimination is the same. Although a patient's disease diagnosis is taken into account when erecting a treatment plan, in TCM as a specific style of Chinese medicine, treatment is primarily based on pattern discrimination.

The benefits of pattern discrimination

If TCM is a safe and non-iatrogenic, holistic medicine, it is entirely because of pattern discrimination. It is pattern discrimination that allows the TCM practitioner to assess the healing virtues of any stimuli on any individual patient. No matter what the patient's disease, if we know that their pattern is one of replete heat, then any food, activity, medicinal, or therapy that adds heat to the body will have a deleterious effect on that specific patient's well-being. If, on the other hand, a person with the same named disease diagnosis had a cool or cold pattern, warming or heating therapies are exactly what he or she requires.

It is this ability to tailor treatment to the exact needs and characteristics of individual patients that makes TCM so safe and non-iatrogenic. The medicinals of Chinese medicine are not safe because they are "herbs." Indeed, many of them are not herbs. They are minerals, chemicals, and animal parts and by-products. Even those that are vegetable in origin are not safe because of that fact. Aconite, Ephedra, and Strychnos are not safe in and of themselves, but are safe only when prescribed to a patient with the right pattern, in the right amount, and for the right period of time. These determinations are not made on the basis of a disease diagnosis but rather on the basis of a TCM pattern discrimination.

TCM is safe medicine when correctly administered based on a professionally correct pattern discrimination, and it is also a holistic medicine. That means it treats the entire person, one's symptoms *and* constitution and one's mind and emotions *as well as* one's body. Thus TCM as a style of Chinese medicine treats disease by restoring balance and harmony to the entire organism. In TCM parlance, it treats the root as well as the branch. In more modern terms, we can say that it treats the figure and the ground. It does not just palliate symptoms, nor does it relieve some symptoms while causing others in the form of side effects.

This ability to treat the whole person and to treat without side effects is entirely based on pattern discrimination. As mentioned above, although even the TCM practitioner starts with a disease diagnosis and does take the disease diagnosis into account when erecting a treatment plan, the main thrust of treatment in TCM is to bring the entire person back into a state of integrated harmony and balance. It is the pattern discrimination that provides the overall picture of the patient's balance and harmony, or lack thereof.

The difference between diseases & patterns

Everyone who is diagnosed as suffering from headache must have, *ipso facto*, pain in the head. But there can be many types of pain in the head: sharp pain, dull pain, pounding pain, slight pain, pain in the temples, pain in the vertex, pain in the forehead, one-sided pain, tight pain, pricking pain, intermittent pain, persistent pain, etc. There can also be many different types of people who have pain in the head: fat people, skinny people, men, women, children, women before menstruation, women after menstruation, women with insomnia, women with somnolence, those with a dry throat and those with excessive mucus, those with a fever and those with chills, those with pale tongues and those with red tongues, or purple tongues, or cracked tongues, or fat tongues, etc.

Every disease has its pathognomonic signs and symptoms. The pathognomonic signs and symptoms of a disease are those that define it. For instance, one cannot be diagnosed as suffering from a headache if one does not have pain or discomfort in the head. Pain in the head can be said to be *the* defining symptom of the disease called headache. However, as we have seen above, different people with the same disease may have all sorts of other, differing signs and symptoms. All patients with the same disease must have certain, pathognomonic symptoms in common. However they may and do have many other symptoms that are different and individualized.

Using the metaphor of figure and ground, we can say that the disease is the figure. Everyone with the same disease has certain same symptoms. The ground, however, is the total pattern. This ground is made up of all the other signs and symptoms that are not necessarily pathognomonic of the diagnosed disease. If one does not see the ground, *i.e.*, the pattern, in which a figure, *i.e.*, the disease, exists, one may give a medicine that should, in theory, treat that disease but that does not work in that particular patient, or worse, may cause side effects or even another disease. This is because the way in which an individual reacts to any medicine or treatment depends not only on the disease process but also on that person's unique constitution.

If TCM therapy is both safe and effective, as it is, it is because we administer treatment based *both* on the disease diagnosis and the patient's overall pattern discrimination. In other words, we tailor our treatment to that patient's exact needs and imbalances, trying to provide just the right stimuli to bring that patient back to balance and thus, a return to health.

How TCM patterns are discriminated

The criteria for establishing a TCM pattern diagnosis are those bits of information gathered by the so-called four examinations (*si zhen*). These are: looking, listening/smelling, questioning, and palpating. Looking means to look with the unaided eyes (except for corrective lenses). The practitioner looks at the patient's eyes, facial complexion, affect, their carriage, gait, and movement, their body type, and at the affected area, for instance looking for erythema, swelling, and bruising in the case of a sprained ankle. Looking also refers to looking at the tongue, its color, shape, presentation, and fur. Smelling and listening as a single verb in Chinese means to smell any body odors or odors of excreta and to listen to the volume and quality of the voice, the sound of respiration, and the sound of coughing or wheezing. Questioning means interrogating the patient about the cause, onset, and signs and symptoms of their complaint and its response to prior treatment; and also asking questions about appetite, thirst, excretions, perspiration, sleep, energy, body warmth, and a number of other body processes, functions, and abilities, such as taste, smell, sight, and hearing. Palpation means feeling the affected area but especially means palpation of the pulse at the radial artery on both wrists.

Although some researchers in the Peoples' Republic of China are beginning to use laboratory analyses to help make or confirm TCM pattern discriminations, until now, TCM patterns are mainly and standardly determined by a combination of signs and symptoms, tongue diagnosis, and pulse diagnosis—all this information having been gathered by means of the four examinations. One pattern is discriminated from another because it differs in its signs and symptoms in whole or in part, or in its tongue diagnosis, or in its pulse diagnosis. For instance, a patient with liver depression, qi stagnation may have lower abdominal distention, premenstrual breast distention, painful menstruation, irritability, a normal colored tongue, and a wiry pulse. Another woman with liver depression, transformative heat might have all the same signs and symptoms but might also have a bitter taste in the mouth, a red tongue with yellow coating, and a wiry, rapid pulse. Yet a third woman might have all the same symptoms as the first but also edema of the four limbs, chilled limbs, fatigue, loose stools when her period comes, night blindness, a pale tongue, and fine and wiry pulse. This patient's pattern is liver depression, spleen and blood vacuity. Thus many patterns may share certain of the same signs and symptoms, but always there will be some difference either in the generalized signs and symptoms, the tongue diagnosis, or the pulse. It is these differences, even though they may be slight, that distinguish one pattern from another.

Types of TCM patterns

In TCM, there are 10 basic systems of pattern discrimination. These are:

1. Five phase pattern discrimination
2. Eight principle pattern discrimination
3. Viscera & bowel pattern discrimination
4. Qi & blood pattern discrimination
5. Fluids & humors pattern discrimination
6. Disease cause pattern discrimination
7. Channel & network vessel pattern discrimination
8. Six aspect pattern discrimination
9. Four aspect pattern discrimination
10. Three burner pattern discrimination

Some of these systems, such as six aspect and four aspect pattern discrimination are relatively complete, self-contained systems that are used for specific types of diseases. However, other of these 10 ways of discriminating patterns are hardly ever used alone but almost always in combination. For instance, if we title a pattern blood vacuity, that pattern is a composite of qi and blood pattern discrimination and eight principle pattern discrimination. If we make a diagnosis of liver blood vacuity, then we have also added viscera and bowel pattern discrimination as well. Thus most patterns described in clinical practice are combinations of several of these systems of pattern discrimination. Liver wood invading spleen earth is a combination of viscera and bowel and five phase pattern discrimination, while damp heat in the liver/gallbladder channels is a combination of disease cause and channel and network vessel pattern discrimination.

It is important to understand that there is no one right way to discriminate a patient's pattern. By this, we mean that five phase pattern discrimination is not better or worse than eight principle pattern discrimination, nor is six aspect pattern discrimination better or worse that four aspect pattern discrimination. Whether a particular system of pattern discrimination is right for a particular patient at hand depends entirely on how well that method of pattern discrimination describes the entirety of that patient's condition. This means that whether a particular pattern discrimination is right or not depends on whether the professionally agreed upon signs and symptoms, tongue, and pulse for that pattern match the patient's.

Books such as this, describing different patterns and their differentiating signs and symptoms, primarily give the simple, standard patterns. However, in actual clinical practice, patients rarely present with such neatly grouped signs and symptoms. This means that in clinical practice, one must combine and tailor these patterns in order to accurately describe the patient's actual situation. In other words, one must modify the patient's pattern until it fits all their signs and symptoms, not try to fit the patient into a nice and neat, simple box that really does not match the entirety of their presentation. In this particular book, we have tried to give many of the commonly seen complicated patterns that actually do present in clinical practice, but even these may require further amendment and modification when dealing with real-life patients. It is important to understand unequivocally that a TCM pattern, whether simple or complex, is a description of the entire patient. It is not like a disease diagnosis, which only describes a fragment of the total presentation—the pathognomonic signs and symptoms of that disease.

How treatment is based on such pattern discrimination

After discriminating between a number of patterns, one next formulates their treatment principles. This is a statement in theory of what needs to be done in order to bring the patient's pattern back to a state of healthy balance. For instance, if a person is suffering from food stagnation with depressive heat, the treatment principles are to disperse food and harmonize the stomach, clear heat and resolve depression. Having formulated those principles, when it comes to internal medicine, the practitioner knows that they should seek a guiding formula from the food-dispersing category. Further, they should seek a formula that also clears heat from the stomach, or they should add appropriate ingredients to the guiding formula in order to clear such heat. Therefore, it is said that the treatment principles are the bridge between the pattern discrimination and the treatment. Knowing the pattern, one formulates the professionally appropriate treatment principles, and these principles should take one immediately to the right category of formulas and medicinals for the patient.

Even if one is using acupuncture and moxibustion instead of internal medicine, the process is basically the same. In this case, every point chosen should accomplish one or more of the stated treatment principles. In TCM, after having written a prescription, be it acupuncture or "herbal," one should be able to rationalize or explain in TCM terms what each point or ingredient is meant to accomplish, and one should not add or do anything that is not explicitly stated or at least obviously inferred by the stated treatment principles. If there is no mention of heat in the patient's pattern and, therefore, no statement of the necessity of clearing heat, there should be no heat-clearing medicinals in the patient's formula unless they are indicated by one of the other treatment principles. In other words, in TCM treatment based on pattern discrimination, we do not "throw in" some points or medicinals without reason. That reason in TCM is always based on returning the patient's *pattern* to a state of balance and harmony and the treatment principles are our guide for accomplishing just that. To do either more or less would result in perpetuating or creating yet another pattern of imbalance.

Viscera & bowel pattern discrimination

In TCM, when it comes to internal damage patterns as opposed to external damage, the main method of pattern discrimination is viscera and bowel pattern discrimination. Therefore, we have focused on viscera and bowel pattern discrimination in this book to the exclusion of almost all external damage patterns. This is not because we are biased against six aspect pattern discrimination, four aspect pattern discrimination, or three burner pattern discrimination. Rather, our focus reflects the nature of our practice as Western practitioners of TCM. Here in the West, most acupuncturists and practitioners of TCM are primarily called upon to treat chronic diseases caused by either internal (*nei yin*) or neither internal nor external causes (*bu nei bu wai yin*). Internal causes refer to internal damage by the seven emotions, while neither internal nor external causes refer to diet, lifestyle, exercise, sex, traumatic injury, parasites, etc. These factors are, in our experience, the major causes of most of the diseases for which most Westerners seek Chinese medical treatment.

Because of the nature of our Western society and our role as caregivers within that society, we are rarely called upon to treat acute, infectious diseases, such as measles, scarlatina, diphtheria, tetanus, cholera, amoebic dysentery, etc. for which six aspect, four aspect, and three burner pattern discrimination were developed. In this book, one will find the treatment of most upper respiratory infections under lung pattern discrimination and the treatment of infectious diarrhea and dysentery under stomach and intestine pattern discrimination. To have added 200 more patterns dealing with six aspect, four aspect, and three burner pattern discrimination would have doubled the size of this book without doubling this book's utility. This is because we believe that the majority of patterns that Western patients present to acupuncturists and practitioners of TCM are included in this book.

However, in stating that we believe that viscera and bowel pattern discrimination is the most important method of TCM pattern discrimination, we do not mean that it is enough to say this or that viscus or bowel is diseased. Rather, one must say in what way that viscus or bowel is out of balance. Therefore, viscera and bowel pattern discrimination is *always* combined with either qi and blood pattern discrimination, fluids and humors pattern discrimination, disease cause pattern discrimination, or eight principle pattern discrimination. In a number of instances, viscera and bowel pattern discrimination implies five phase discrimination even though five phase terminology is not specifically used. For instance, liver invading the stomach can also be described as wood invading earth. However, liver invading the stomach is more specific and names exactly which earth organ is affected by this invasion. In some cases, the terminology of liver wood invading spleen earth is used. In those cases, the author is indicating five phase theory and the *ke* or restraint cycle while also specifying exactly which organ within earth is affected.

Conclusion

It is the authors' belief that the single greatest thing that TCM has to offer to the Western world is treatment based on pattern discrimination. Yes, acupuncture is a wonderfully effective therapy, as is *Tui Na* or Chinese medical massage. Yes, Astragalus, Lycium berries, Ginseng, Cordyceps, Ganoderma, and Polyporus are all wonderful Chinese medicinals. But TCM as a style of Chinese medicine is not really defined by its therapeutic modalities and pharmaceuticals. After all, many of these are not native Chinese but rather imports as is, for instance, American Ginseng.

If one understands treatment based on pattern discrimination, one can apply this methodology to any medicinal or any therapeutic modality originating anywhere in the world. It is this methodology of basing treatment on pattern discrimination that is, we believe, Chinese medicine's most important gift to the world. It is a way of seeing a person in their entirety and of basing treatment on that whole person.

1
Viscera & Bowel Pattern Discrimination

Liver & Gallbladder Patterns

Liver Depression, Qi Stagnation

Disease causes, disease mechanisms: Emotional stress, anger, and frustration cause the liver to lose its control over coursing and discharge. This hampers the liver's orderly reaching and thus the movement of qi is not smoothly flowing. Instead it accumulates in areas of the body associated with the liver or traversed by channels and vessels connected with the liver.

Main symptoms: Irritability, mental depression, chest, lateral costal, breast, and abdominal distention and oppression, sighing, dysmenorrhea, irregular menstruation

Tongue & coating: A normal tongue or a slightly darkish tongue with thin, white tongue coating

Pulse image: Wiry

Treatment principles: Course the liver and rectify the qi

Rx: *Chai Hu Shu Gan San* (Bupleurum Soothe the Liver Powder)

Ingredients:

Pericarpium Citri Reticulatae (*Chen Pi*)
Radix Bupleuri (*Chai Hu*)
Radix Ligustici Wallichii (*Chuan Xiong*)
Fructus Aurantii (*Zhi Ke*)
Radix Albus Paeoniae Lactiflorae (*Bai Shao*)
mix-fried Radix Glycyrrhizae (*Zhi Gan Cao*)
Rhizoma Cyperi Rotundi (*Xiang Fu*)

Additions & subtractions: For breast distension and pain, add Tuber Curcumae (*Yu Jin*). For palpable lumps in the breast, add Semen Citri Reticulatae (*Ju He*), Fructus Liquidambaris Taiwaniae (*Lu Lu Tong*), and Squama Manitis Pentadactylis (*Chuan Shan Jia*). For dysmenorrhea, add Rhizoma Corydalis (*Yan Hu Suo*).

Acupuncture & moxibustion: *Tai Chong* (Liv 3), *He Gu* (LI 4)

Auxiliary points: Add *Shan Zhong* (CV 17) for chest and breast distention and pain. Add *Qi Hai* (CV 6) for lower abdominal distention and pain. Add *Qi Min* (Liv 14) for hypochondral distention and pain. Add *Zhong Wan* (CV 12) for epigastric fullness and distention.

Key advice: Although this pattern is extremely important, it is rarely met with as a discreet, single pattern in clinical practice. Because of the interrelationships between the liver and spleen and the qi and blood, when there is liver depression, qi stagnation, typically there is also concomitant spleen vacuity and blood vacuity. Thus the signs and symptoms are variable. The wiry pulse is probably the single most important sign in identifying this pattern. For its remedy, patients must usually be counselled on getting regular exercise, deep relaxation, and stress reduction.

Liver Qi Counterflowing Upward

Disease causes, disease mechanisms: If, due to stress, anger, and frustration, the liver loses control over coursing and discharge and its orderly reaching is inhibited, qi does not move but rather stagnates and accumulates. Because qi is yang, it tends to move upward. Thus when liver qi accumulates, it often counterflows upward.

Main symptoms: Periumbilical palpitations followed by an up-surging of qi from the abdomen to the sternum when the patient becomes upset, cold limbs and body when nervous but restoration of the heat in the limbs when relaxed and at ease, heart palpitations

Tongue & coating: A white, slimy tongue coating

Pulse image: A wiry pulse that tends to be hooked. This means that pulses in the inch or *cun* positions lack root.

Treatment principles: Level the liver and downbear upward counterflow

Rx: *Ben Tun Wan* (Running Piglet Pill)

Ingredients:

Fructus Meliae Toosendan (*Chuan Lian Zi*)
Sclerotium Poriae Cocos (*Fu Ling*)
Semen Citri Reticulatae (*Ju He*)
Semen Litchi Chinensis (*Li Zhi He*)
Fructus Foeniculi Vulgaris (*Xiao Hui Xiang*)
Radix Auklandiae (*Mu Xiang*)

Acupuncture & moxibustion: *Tai Chong* (Liv 3), *Shan Zhong* (CV 17), *Nei Guan* (Per 6), *Gong Sun* (Sp 4)

Key advice: In its simple, discreet form, this pattern is also not commonly met in clinical practice. However, it often does form part of the core mechanism for more complicated patterns frequently seen in Western patients.

Liver Qi Invading the Stomach

Disease causes, disease mechanisms: Due to internal damage by the seven affects, the liver may become depressed and then invade the stomach causing loss of harmony of the stomach qi. Thus the stomach qi counterflows upward.

Main symptoms: Epigastric and lateral costal distention and pain, nausea, vomiting, hiccup, burping and belching

Tongue & coating: A normal tongue with a thin, white coating

Pulse image: A wiry pulse, especially in the right bar or *guan* position

Treatment principles: Course the liver and rectify the qi, harmonize the stomach and downbear counterflow

Rx: *Xuan Fu Dai Zhe Tang* (Inula & Hematite Decoction)

Ingredients:

Flos Inulae (*Xuan Fu Hua*)
Haemititum (*Dai Zhe Shi*)
Radix Panacis Ginseng (*Ren Shen*)
Rhizoma Pinelliae Ternatae (*Ban Xia*)
uncooked Rhizoma Zingiberis (*Sheng Jiang*)
mix-fried Radix Glycyrrhizae (*Zhi Gan Cao*)
Fructus Zizyphi Jujubae (*Da Zao*)

Additions & subtractions: This formula is for the combined pattern of liver qi invading the stomach with an element of spleen vacuity, dampness, and phlegm. If there is no spleen vacuity, one can subtract the Ginseng, mix-fried Licorice, and Red Dates. If there is phlegm dampness as evidenced by a slimy tongue coating, add Cortex Magnoliae Officinalis (*Hou Po*), Sclerotium Poriae Cocos (*Fu Ling*), and Pericarpium Citri Reticulatae (*Chen Pi*).

Acupuncture & moxibustion: *Tai Chong* (Liv 3), *Nei Guan* (Per 6), *Zhong Wan* (CV 12), *Zu San Li* (St 36)

Auxiliary points: If there is phlegm dampness, add *Pi Shu* (Bl 20), *Wei Shu* (Bl 21), *Feng Long* (St 40), and *Shang Qiu* (Sp 5).

Key advice: In most cases, there will be an element of spleen vacuity and dampness if not phlegm. Because of the close interrelationships between these three viscera and bowels, if one becomes affected, they all frequently become involved, especially if the precipitating cause is liver depression, qi stagnation.

Liver Depression, Spleen Vacuity

Disease causes, disease mechanisms: Due to stress, anger, and frustration, the liver may lose its orderly reaching. In that case, stagnant qi accumulates. Eventually, it will counterflow to attack the spleen according to the five phase control cycle. This is especially likely if the patient habitually indulges in sweets in an attempt to relax the liver. This weakens the spleen and makes it all the riper for predation. Because the spleen is the latter heaven or postnatal source for the engenderment and transformation of blood, spleen vacuity may result in liver blood vacuity, which then only worsens the qi stagnation. This is because blood is the mother of qi and the blood softens and harmonizes the liver.

Main symptoms: Liver depression signs and symptoms as described above, such as menstrual irregularity and breast distention, plus spleen vacuity symptoms such as fatigued spirit, reduced appetite, loose stools, fatigue, and lack of strength

Tongue & coating: A pale, somewhat darkish tongue which is typically swollen and has the indentations of the teeth on its edges and a thin, white coating

Pulse image: Wiry and fine

Treatment principles: Coarse the liver and resolve depression, fortify the spleen and harmonize the constructive

Rx: *Xiao Yao San* (Rambling Powder)

Ingredients:

Radix Bupleuri (*Chai Hu*)
Radix Angelicae Sinensis (*Dang Gui*)
Radix Albus Paeoniae Lactiflorae (*Bai Shao*)
Rhizoma Atractylodis Macrocephalae (*Bai Zhu*)
Sclerotium Poriae Cocos (*Fu Ling*)
mix-fried Radix Glycyrrhizae (*Zhi Gan Cao*)
Herba Menthae (*Bo He*)
uncooked Rhizoma Zingiberis (*Sheng Jiang*)

Additions & subtractions: For concomitant qi vacuity, add Radix Panacis Ginseng (*Ren Shen*) or Radix Codonopsis Pilosulae (*Dang Shen*) and Radix Astragali Membranacei (*Huang Qi*). In women with qi vacuity, one can consider adding Radix Codonopsis Pilosulae (*Dang Shen*) and Radix Pseudostellariae (*Tai Zi Shen*). For qi vacuity and spleen weakness with borborygmus and loose stools, subtract Mint and add Rhizoma Atractylodis (*Cang Zhu*), Rhizoma Cimicifugae (*Sheng Ma*), and Pericarpium Citri Reticulatae (*Chen Pi*).

Acupuncture & moxibustion: *Tai Chong* (Liv 3), *He Gu* (LI 4), *Zu San Li* (St 36), *San Yin Jiao* (Sp 6)

Auxiliary points: Add *Pi Shu* (Bl 20), *Wei Shu* (Bl 21), and *Tian Shu* (St 25) for loose stools. Add *Ge Shu* (Bl 17), *Gan Shu* (Bl 18), and *Pi Shu* (Bl 20) for blood vacuity.

Key advice: This combined pattern is commonly encountered in clinical practice. There is the wiry pulse of liver depression and some signs of qi accumulation like breast distention, but there are also symptoms of spleen qi vacuity, such as fatigue and, typically, loose stools.

Some Chinese doctors recognize a liver qi vacuity pattern. However, in reviewing the literature on this pattern, the authors believe this is nothing other than a slight variation of the pattern discussed above: liver depression, spleen vacuity. Chen Jia-xu and Yang Wei-yi give the symptoms of liver qi vacuity as fatigue, shortness of breath, spontaneous sweating, depression, worry, or agitation, profuse dreaming, tendency to fear, chest and lateral costal fullness and oppression, frequent sighing, lower abdominal distention, irregular menstruation, dysmenorrhea, amenorrhea, a pale, fat, swollen tongue with possible teeth marks on its edges, and a vacuous, forceless pulse. These symptoms are a combination of liver depression, qi stagnation symptoms and generalized qi vacuity symptoms. Although one might interpret some of these vacuity symptoms as lung or heart qi vacuity symptoms, since the spleen is the postnatal root of qi and blood engenderment and transformation, we see no need to create a liver depression lung qi vacuity pattern. This is especially so when one sees that the treatment principles given by Chen & Yang are to supplement the qi and emolliate the liver, soothe the liver and replenish the spleen. The formula given is *Yang Gan Yi Qi Jian* (Nourish the Liver & Boost the Qi Decoction): Radix Astragali Membranacei (*Huang Qi*), Radix Bupleuri (*Chai Hu*), Fructus Aurantii (*Zhi Ke*), Pericarpium Citri Reticulatae (*Chen Pi*), mix-fried Radix Glycyrrhizae (*Zhi Gan Cao*), Radix Angelicae Sinensis (*Dang Gui*), and Radix Albus Paeoniae Lactiflorae (*Bai Shao*). For another variation on this same pattern, the reader should see heart/gallbladder qi vacuity below.

Liver Depression, Transformative Heat

Disease causes, disease mechanisms: If due to stress, anger, or frustration, the liver becomes depressed and the qi becomes stagnant, qi will accumulate. Because qi is yang, it is inherently warm. If enough qi becomes depressed and stagnant it will transform from just qi stagnation to depressive heat. Thus there are the signs and symptoms of liver depression mixed with those of heat. In addition, depressive heat may force the blood to move recklessly outside its pathways.

Main symptoms: Irascibility, easy anger, impetuosity, chest oppression, heart vexation, mental restlessness, insomnia, excessive dreams, red eyes, a red facial complexion, acne, heart palpitations, breast distention but more prominent pain and hypersensitivity and pain of the nipples, a bitter taste in the mouth, oral thirst, early menstruation, excessive menstruation, or flooding and leaking

Tongue & coating: A dark red tongue or dark red and/or swollen tongue edges with a thin, yellow coating

Pulse image: Wiry and rapid

Treatment principles: Course the liver and rectify the qi, clear heat and resolve depression

Rx: *Dan Zhi Xiao Yao San* (Moutan & Gardenia Rambling Powder)

Ingredients:

Fructus Gardeniae Jasminoidis (*Shan Zhi Zi*)
Cortex Radicis Moutan (*Mu Dan Pi*)
Radix Bupleuri (*Chai Hu*)
Radix Angelicae Sinensis (*Dang Gui*)
Radix Albus Paeoniae Lactiflorae (*Bai Shao*)
Rhizoma Atractylodes Macrocephalae (*Bai Zhu*)
Sclerotium Poriae Cocos (*Fu Ling*)
Radix Glycyrrhizae (*Gan Cao*)
Herba Menthae Haplocalycis (*Bo He*)

Additions & subtractions: For a red face, heart vexation, and easy anger, add Rhizoma Coptidis Chinensis (*Huang Lian*) and Radix Gentianae Scabrae (*Long Dan Cao*). For acne, add Radix Scutellariae Baicalensis (*Huang Qin*). For early or excessive menstruation or for flooding and leaking, add Radix Scutellariae Baicalensis (*Huang Qin*) and Radix Sanguisorbae (*Di Yu*). For epistaxis, hemoptysis, or hematemesis, add Radix Scutellariae Baicalensis (*Huang Qi*) and Radix Rubiae Cordifoliae (*Qian Cao*). For breast pain and nipple soreness, add Herba Cum Radice Taraxaci Mongolici (*Pu Gong Ying*) and Spica Prunellae Vulgaris (*Xia Ku Cao*).

Acupuncture & moxibustion: *Xiang Jian* (Liv 2) through-and-through to *Tai Chong* (Liv 3), *He Gu* (LI 4), and *Qu Chi* (LI 11), *Da Ling* (Per 7), *Xin Shu* (Bl 15), *Gan Shu* (Bl 18)

Auxiliary points: If there is heart vexation, heart palpitations, insomnia, or excessive dreams, add *Da Ling* (Per 7) and *Xin Shu* (Bl 15). If there is bleeding due to blood heat, add *Xue Hai* (Sp 10) and *Da Dun* (Liv 1). If that blood is menstrual bleeding, add *San Yin Jiao* (Sp 6) and *Zhong Ji* (CV 3).

Key advice: This is also a very commonly met with pattern in clinical practice. Its key discriminating points are that the pulse is wiry *and* fast and there is a bitter taste in the mouth. However, this bitter taste is often only present upon arising in the morning.

Liver/Stomach Depressive Heat & Counterflow

Disease causes, disease mechanisms: If, due to stress, the liver becomes depressed and the qi becomes stagnant and accumulates, it may counterflow horizontally to invade the stomach. This causes loss of harmony of the stomach and upward counterflow of stomach qi. However, in most cases, there is not just counterflow but also depressive heat in both the liver and stomach.

Main symptoms: Lateral costal pain, indeterminate gnawing hunger, epigastric focal distention, nausea, vomiting, hiccup, belching, acid regurgitation

Tongue & coating: A red tongue with a yellow coating

Pulse image: A wiry, rapid pulse

Treatment principles: Clear the liver and stomach, resolve depression and downbear counterflow, harmonize the stomach and stop vomiting

Rx: *Zuo Jin Wan* (Left Metal Pills)

Ingredients:

Rhizoma Coptidis Chinensis (*Huang Lian*)
Fructus Evodiae Rutecarpae (*Wu Zhu Yu*)

Additions & subtractions: For severe distension, add Fructus Meliae Toosendan (*Chuan Lian Zi*). For pronounced acid regurgitation, add Os Sepiae Seu Sepiellae (*Hai Piao Xiao*) and Concha Arcae (*Wa Leng Zi*). This two-ingredient formula is often added to other formulas when upward counterflow and depressive heat of the liver and stomach complicate other patterns.

Acupuncture & moxibustion: *Zhong Wan* (CV 12), *Nei Guan* (Per 6), *Tai Chong* (Liv 3) or *Xiang Jian* (Liv 2), *Nei Ting* (St 44)

Auxiliary points: For vomiting, hiccup, and acid regurgitation, add *Wei Shu* (Bl 21) and *Zu San Li* (St 36).

Key advice: This pattern is a subpattern of the previous one and, therefore, they share the same or similar tongue and pulse images. In actual clinical practice, one often finds liver/stomach depressive heat with spleen vacuity. In that case, the signs of heat in the stomach may only be increased appetite and facial acne along the *yang ming*. If there is acid regurgitation, this symptom points to heat as opposed to simple belching or hiccup being only counterflowing qi.

Liver Wind Stirring Internally

Disease causes, disease mechanisms: This is a more serious progression from qi counterflow, which, as we have seen, is mainly due to internal damage by the seven affects. Once again, qi stagnation has accumulated to the point where it counterflows upward. In the case of qi counterflow, the condition tends to be chronic and aggravated by stressful episodes. In the case of liver wind stirring internally, upward counterflow tends to be both more serious and more constant. If really serious it leads to syncope.

Main symptoms: Headache, dizziness, vertigo, distention of the eyes, tinnitus, hot pain in the brain region, vexatious heat within the heart, a tidal red facial complexion, frequent belching, inability to control the limbs of the body, deviation of the eyes and mouth, if serious, dizziness and vertigo leading to collapse, loss of consciousness of human affairs, essence spirit diminished and scanty

Tongue & coating: A red with a dryish, somewhat yellowish tongue coating

Pulse image: A long, wiry, forceful pulse

Treatment principles: Settle the liver and extinguish wind, enrich yin and subdue yang

Rx: *Zhen Gan Xi Feng Tang* (Settle the Liver & Extinguish Wind Decoction)

Ingredients:

Radix Achyranthis Bidentatae (*Huai Niu Xi*)
Haemititum (*Dai Zhe Shi*)
uncooked Os Draconis (*Sheng Long Gu*)
uncooked Concha Ostreae (*Sheng Mu Li*)
uncooked Plastrum Testudinis (*Shen Gui Ban*)
uncooked Radix Albus Paeoniae Lactiflorae (*Sheng Bai Hang Yao*)
Radix Scrophulariae Ningpoensis (*Yuan Shen*)
Tuber Asparagi Cochinensis (*Tian Dong*)
Fructus Meliae Toosendan (*Chuan Lian Zi*)
uncooked Fructus Germinatus Hordei Vulgaris (*Sheng Mai Ya*)
Herba Artemisiae Capillaris (*Yin Chen*)
Radix Glycyrrhizae (*Gan Cao*)

Additions & subtractions: For headache, blurred vision, vertigo, and dizziness, add Spica Prunellae Vulgaris (*Xia Ku Cao*) and Flos Chrysanthemi Morifolii (*Ju Hua*). For excessive phlegm, subtract Licorice and Scrophularia and add bile-processed Rhizoma Arisaematis (*Dan Nan Xing*) and Bulbus Fritillariae Cirrhosae (*Chuan Bei Mu*). If there is concomitant kidney vacuity, add prepared Radix Rehmanniae (*Shu Di*) and Fructus Corni Officinalis (*Shan Zhu Yu*).

Acupuncture & moxibustion: *Gan Shu* (Bl 18), *Tai Chong* (Liv 3), *Feng Chi* (GB 20), *Yang Ling Quan* (GB 34), *Qu Chi* (LI 11)

Auxiliary points: For headache, dizziness, and vertigo, add *Bai Hui* (GV 20) and *Yin Tang* (M-HN-3).

Key advice: This pattern is a type of qi counterflow in turn due to qi stagnation. However, in this pattern, yang is hyperactive above and yin is vacuous below. Usually this is due to long-term liver depression and qi stagnation with consequent enduring blood vacuity that has eventually consumed and damaged yin. It should be kept in mind that internally engendered wind is nothing other than yang qi counterflowing upward and outward.

Insufficiency of Liver Blood

Disease causes, disease mechanisms: Due to extreme or repeated blood loss, constitutional kidney yin vacuity, or spleen weakness and deficiency, there is insufficient blood stored in the liver. This results in symptoms of insufficient nourishment of the tissues and functions associated with the liver.

Main symptoms: A somber white or sallow yellow facial complexion, dizziness, heart palpitations, pale lips and nails, blurred vision, night blindness, insomnia, lateral costal pain, twitching of the muscles, numbness of the limbs, scanty, delayed, or blocked menstruation (*i.e.*, amenorrhea)

Tongue & coating: A pale tongue with a thin, white coating

Pulse image: A fine, wiry pulse

Treatment principles: Supplement the liver and nourish the blood

Rx: *Bu Gan Tang* (Supplement the Liver Decoction)

Ingredients:

Radix Angelicae Sinensis (*Dang Gui*)
Radix Ligustici Wallichii (*Chuan Xiong*)
Radix Albus Paeoniae Lactiflorae (*Bai Shao*)
prepared Radix Rehmanniae (*Shu Di Huang*)
Semen Zizyphi Spinosae (*Suan Zao Ren*)
Fructus Chaenomelis Lagenariae (*Mu Gua*)
mix-fried Radix Glycyrrhizae (*Zhi Gan Cao*)

Additions & subtractions: The formula above treats liver blood vacuity with both insomnia and tremors and numbness of the extremities. If there is mainly menstrual irregularity, one can use the first four ingredients (*i.e.*, *Si Wu Tang* [Four Materials Decoction]) with any of a large number of additions. For instance, if there are simultaneous symptoms of qi stagnation, one can add Rhizoma Cyperi Rotundi (*Xiang Fu*) and Radix Bupleuri (*Chai Hu*). If there is concomitant spleen qi vacuity, add Radix Astragali Membranacei (*Huang Qi*) and Radix Panacis Ginseng (*Ren Shen*) or Radix Codonopsis Pilosulae (*Dang Shen*). For a large list of modifications of *Si Wu Tang*, see Bob Flaws' *How to Write a* TCM *Herbal Formula* or his *Seventy Essential* TCM *Formulas for Beginners*.

Acupuncture & moxibustion: *San Yin Jiao* (Sp 6), *Gan Shu* (Bl 18), *Pi Shu* (Bl 20), *Ge Shu* (Bl 17), *Zu San Li* (St 36)

Auxiliary points: If liver blood vacuity is due more to kidney yin vacuity than to spleen qi vacuity, remove *Pi Shu* and *Zu San Li* and add *Shen Shu* (Bl 23) and *Qu Quan* (Liv 8). If there is menstrual irregularity, add *Guan Yuan* (CV 4). If there are heart palpitations and insomnia, add *Nei Guan* (Per 6) and *Shen Men* (Ht 7).

Key advice: Liver depression/qi stagnation and liver blood vacuity commonly occur together. This is because, on the one hand, the blood is the mother of the qi. Blood vacuity therefore results in impairment of the liver's function of coursing and discharging. On the other hand, liver depression is often complicated by spleen vacuity and the spleen is the latter heaven source of blood engenderment and transformation. This is why *Xiao Yao San* (Rambling Powder) has within it medicinals to both nourish the blood and fortify the spleen.

Liver Blood Insufficiency Engendering Wind

Disease causes, disease mechanisms: Blood is the mother of qi, if blood becomes insufficient due once again to loss, spleen qi vacuity, or kidney yin vacuity, yang qi may counterflow upward and outward. Lack of blood to nourish the sinews gives rise to symptoms of contraction and spasm, while stirring of wind gives rise to symptoms of involuntary movement, such as tremors and convulsions.

Main symptoms: A somber white or sallow yellow facial complexion, pale lips and nails, tremors and numbness of the limbs, convulsions, and opistothonus

Tongue & coating: A pale tongue with a thin, white coating

Pulse image: A fine, wiry pulse

Treatment principles: Supplement the liver, nourish the blood, and dispel wind

Rx: *Si Wu Tang Jia Wei* (Four Materials Decoction with Added Flavors)

Ingredients:

Radix Angelicae Sinensis (*Dang Gui*)
Radix Albus Paeoniae Lactiflorae (*Bai Shao*)

prepared Radix Rehmanniae (*Shu Di*)
Radix Ligustici Wallichii (*Chuan Xiong*)
Radix Gentianae Macrophyllae (*Qin Jiao*)
Radix Et Rhizoma Notopterygii (*Qiang Huo*)

Acupuncture & moxibustion: San Yin Jiao (*Sp 6*), *Zu San Li* (St 36), *Ge Shu* (Bl 17), *Gan Shu* (Bl 18), *Pi Shu* (Bl 20), *Bai Hui* (GV 20), *Feng Chi* (GB 20)

Key advice: Many books do not list a separate liver wind due to blood vacuity pattern, since, in most cases of internal stirring of liver wind, there are symptoms of blood *and* yin vacuity *with* either vacuity or replete heat. In clinical practice, one can sometimes see this simpler pattern in women who experience dizziness and numbness after menstruation.

Replete Fire in the Liver Channel

Disease causes, disease mechanisms: This may be due to emotional stress, frustration, and anger causing enduring depression, which then transforms into heat. If exacerbated by a bout of intense anger or stress, this heat may become fire that flares upward, affecting the areas of the head connected with the liver and its associated channels and network vessels. It may also be caused by overeating hot, acrid, peppery foods, alcohol, and greasy, fatty, thick-flavored foods. These may give rise to dampness, which pours downward to the liver channel in the lower burner and may cause heat in that channel. This then results in damp heat in the liver channel in the lower burner.

Main symptoms: 1) Liver fire flaring upward: Headache, red eyes, lateral costal pain, a bitter taste in the mouth, loss of hearing, swelling of the ears; 2) Damp heat in the liver channel: Genital swelling, genital itching, impotence, genital sweating, urinary strangury, turbid urine, damp heat abnormal vaginal discharge in women

Tongue & coating: A red tongue with slimy, yellow coating

Pulse image: A rapid, forceful or rapid, slippery, wiry pulse

Treatment principles: 1) Clear the liver and drain fire; 2) clear heat and disinhibit dampness

Rx: *Long Dan Xie Gan Tang* (Gentiana Drain the Liver Decoction)

Ingredients:

Radix Gentianae Scabrae (*Long Dan Cao*)
Radix Scutellariae Baicalensis (*Huang Qin*)
Fructus Gardeniae Jasminoidis (*Shan Zhi Zi*)

Rhizoma Alismatis (*Ze Xie*)
Caulis Akebiae (*Mu Tong*)
Semen Plantaginis (*Che Qian Zi*)
Radix Angelicae Sinensis (*Dang Gui*)
raw Radix Rehmanniae (*Sheng Di*)
Radix Bupleuri (*Chai Hu*)
uncooked Radix Glycyrrhizae (*Sheng Gan Cao*)

Additions & subtractions: In case of acute icteric hepatitis, subtract Alisma and Plantago and add Herba Artemisiae Capillaris (*Yin Chen*). For a reddish vaginal discharge and a wiry, rapid pulse, add Radix Rubrus Paeoniae Lactiflorae (*Chi Shao*) and Stamen Nelumbinis Nuciferae (*Lian Xu*). For severe headache and red, painful eyes, add Flos Chrysanthemi Morifolli (*Ju Hua*) and Folium Mori Albi (*Sang Ye*). For hemoptysis due to liver fire damaging the lungs, add Cortex Radicis Moutan (*Dan Pi*) and Cacumen Biotae Orientalis (*Ce Bai Ye*).

Acupuncture & moxibustion: *Yang Ling Quan* (GB 34), *Xing Jian* (Liv 2) through-and-through to *Tai Chong* (Liv 3), *Gan Shu* (Bl 18), *San Yin Jiao* (Sp 6), *Ying Ling Quan* (Sp 9)

Auxiliary points: Add local points in either the areas of the eyes, ears, and head or the genitalia.

Key advice: There are actually two different patterns here: 1) liver fire flaring upward and 2) damp heat in the liver channel. However, because both these patterns are treated with the same basic medicinal formula, they are presented under the more general terminology of replete fire in the liver channel. Students should be cautioned, however, that, at least with Western patients, *Long Dan Xie Gan Tang* is not all that frequently prescribed a formula. This is because most Western patients have mixed repletion/vacuity conditions and especially damaged spleens. In such cases, this formula is too bitter and cold and damages the spleen and stomach even more.

Liver Fire Attacking the Lungs

Disease causes, disease mechanisms: Liver fire due to emotional stress and anger may not only flare upward to affect the eyes, ears, and head in general, but it may also damage the network vessels of the lungs. In this case, extreme heat causes the blood to move recklessly outside its pathways, resulting in bloody phlegm and hemoptysis.

Main symptoms: Bloody phlegm accompanied by cough, hemoptysis, coughing and wheezing, fever with skin that feels hot to the touch, all of which worsen in the late afternoon. There may also be a dry mouth and little or difficult-to-expectorate phlegm.

Tongue & coating: A red tongue with a yellow coating

Pulse image: A fine, wiry, rapid pulse

Treatment principles: Clear heat from liver and lungs, cool the blood and stop bleeding, calm wheezing

Rx: *Xie Bai San* (Drain the White Powder)

Ingredients:

Cortex Radicis Mori Albi (*Sang Bai Pi*)
Cortex Radicis Lycii Chinensis (*Di Gu Pi*)
mix-fried Radix Glycyrrhizae (*Zhi Gan Cao*)
Semen Oryzae Sativae (*Geng Mi*)

Additions & subtractions: For hemoptysis and bloody phlegm, add Rhizoma Bletillae Striatae (*Bai Ji*) and Cacumen Biotae Orientalis (*Ce Bai Ye*). In order to protect the spleen and stomach more effectively, remove the Polished Rice and add Sclerotium Poriae Cocos (*Fu Ling*). For more severe heat, add Radix Scutellariae Baicalensis (*Huang Qin*) and Radix Anemarrhenae (*Zhi Mu*).

Acupuncture & moxibustion: *Gan Shu* (Bl 18), *Fei Shu* (Bl 13), *Chi Ze* (Lu 5), *Xing Jian* (Liv 2), *Yu Ji* (Lu 10)

Key advice: Either liver depressive heat or liver fire may rise up to the lungs. Liver/lung depressive heat results in cough and acne, while liver fire results in hemoptysis and bloody phlegm. In this case, liver fire is a more serious evolution of depressive heat. The pulse is not only wiry and fast but also fine because heat has damaged lung yin.

Liver Fire Attacking the Stomach

Disease causes, disease mechanisms: Just as depressive liver heat may attack the stomach so may liver fire. In this case, fire damages the network vessels of the stomach, thus causing hematemesis.

Main symptoms: Epigastric pain, hematemesis, acid eructation

Tongue & coating: A red tongue with yellow coating

Pulse image: A rapid, wiry pulse

Treatment principles: Drain liver/stomach fire, cool the blood and stop bleeding, stop vomiting

Rx: *Huang Lian Jie Du Tang* (Coptis Resolve Toxins Decoction) plus *Si Sheng Wan* (Four Uncooked Pills)

Ingredients:

Rhizoma Coptidis Chinensis (*Huang Lian*)
Cortex Phellodendri (*Huang Bai*)
Radix Scutellariae Baicalensis (*Huang Qin*)
Fructus Gardeniae Jasminoidis (*Shan Zhi Zi*)
uncooked Radix Rehmanniae (*Sheng Di*)
uncooked Cacumen Biotae Orientalis (*Ce Bai Ye*)
uncooked Folium Nelumbinis Nuciferae (*He Ye*)
uncooked Artemisiae Argyii (*Ai Ye*)

Acupuncture & moxibustion: *Tai Chong* (Liv 3), *Nei Ting* (St 44), *Gan Shu* (Bl 18), *Wei Shu* (Bl 21), *Zhong Wan* (CV 12), *Nei Guan* (Per 6)

Liver Yang Vacuity

Disease causes, disease mechanisms: Enduring fright or mental depression may consume yang qi. This is because the liver's orderly reaching and control over coursing and discharge are empowered by kidney yang's steaming and warming.

Main symptoms: Emotional depression, anxiety and proneness to fear, blurred vision, bodily cold, a dark facial complexion, impotence in men or clear, chilly vaginal discharge in women, infertility in women, and sterility in men

Tongue & coating: A pale tongue with a white coating and a possibly red tip

Pulse image: A deep, fine, wiry, slow pulse or, more commonly in Western patients, a surging, floating, forceless pulse in the inch position with a floating, fine, and wiry left cubit position

Treatment principles: For fright, supplement the liver and gallbladder, strengthen yang, and quiet the spirit. For impotence, supplement the liver and strengthen yang. For fatigue, warm yang and nourish the liver, supplement the qi and fortify the spleen. For females, supplement and nourish the qi and blood, regulate and rectify the *chong* and *ren*.

Rx: *Wen Jing Tang* (Warm the Menses Decoction)

Ingredients:

Fructus Evodiae Rutacarpae (*Wu Zhu Yu*)
Ramulus Cinnamomi Cassiae (*Gui Zhi*)
Radix Angelicae Sinensis (*Dang Gui*)
Radix Ligustici Wallichii (*Chuan Xiong*)
Radix Albus Paeoniae Lactiflorae (*Bai Shao*)
Gelatinum Corii Asini (*E Jiao*)
Tuber Ophiopogonis Japonici (*Mai Men Dong*)
Cortex Radicis Moutan (*Mu Dan Pi*)
Radix Panacis Ginseng (*Ren Shen*)
Radix Glycyrrhizae Uralensis (*Gan Cao*)
uncooked Rhizoma Zingiberis (*Sheng Jiang*)
Rhizoma Pinelliae Ternatae (*Ban Xia*)

Additions & subtractions: For concomitant qi stagnation, add Rhizoma Cyperi Rotundi (*Xiang Fu*) and Radix Linderae Strychnifoliae (*Wu Yao*). For more severe lower abdominal cold and pain, omit Ophiopogon and Moutan and add Fructus Foeniculi Vulgaris (*Xiao Hui Xiang*) and Folium Artemisiae Argyii (*Ai Ye*). In addition, substitute Cortex Cinnamomi (*Rou Gui*) for Ramulus Cinnamomi.

Acupuncture & moxibustion: *Xin Shu* (Bl 15), *Gan Shu* (Bl 18), *Shen Shu* (Bl 23), *Ming Men* (GV 4), *Zu San Li* (St 36), *San Yin Jiao* (Sp 6), *Shen Que* (CV 8)

Key advice: Most books on TCM pattern discrimination do not include this pattern. That is because it is actually more complex than its name appears. It consists of liver blood vacuity, spleen qi vacuity, and kidney yang vacuity with upward counterflow of yang qi. Because of vacuity cold, there may also be a complicating factor of blood stasis. This pattern is commonly seen in women with perimenopausal complaints. Due to the pervasive stress in Western society and the prevalence of patients with counterflow conditions, this pattern is a good one to know.

Hyperactivity of Liver Yang

Disease causes, disease mechanisms: Enduring stress may cause enduring liver depression, transformative heat. This depressive heat consumes and damages blood and eventually yin. Yin becomes too weak to control yang, and yang counterflows upward with symptoms of heat and repletion above but symptoms of cold and vacuity below.

Main symptoms: Headache, dizziness, vertigo, insomnia, paralysis or convulsions, deviation of the mouth and eyes

Tongue & coating: A red tongue

Pulse image: A wiry, rapid pulse

Treatment principles: Level the liver and extinguish the wind, clear heat and quicken the blood, supplement and boost the liver and kidneys

Rx: *Tian Ma Gou Teng Yin* (Gastrodia & Uncaria Drink)

Ingredients:

Rhizoma Gastrodiae Elatae (*Tian Ma*)
Ramulus Uncariae Cum Uncis (*Gou Teng*)
Concha Haliotidis (*Shi Jue Ming*)
Fructus Gardeniae Jasminoidis (*Shan Zhi Zi*)
Radix Scutellariae Baicalensis (*Huang Qin*)
Radix Cyathulae (*Chuan Niu Xi*)
Cortex Eucommiae Ulmoidis (*Du Zhong*)
Herba Leonuri Heterophylli (*Yi Mu Cao*)
Ramulus Loranthi Seu Visci (*Sang Ji Sheng*)
Caulis Polygoni Multiflori (*Ye Jiao Teng*)
Cinnabar(-processed) Sclerotium Pararadicis Poriae Cocos (*Zhu Fu Shen*)

Additions & subtractions: If there are dizziness and vertigo or head distention, add Spica Prunellae Vulgaris (*Xia Ku Cao*) and Flos Chrysanthemi Morifolii (*Ju Hua*). If the disease is serious, add Cornu Antelopis Saiga-tatarici (*Ling Yang Jiao*). If there is numbness of the extremities, add Caulis Milletiae Seu Spatholobi (*Jie Xue Teng*) and Lumbricus (*Di Long*).

Acupuncture & moxibustion: *Bai Hui* (GV 20), *Yin Tang* (M-HN-3), *Feng Chi* (GB 20), *Tai Chong* (Liv 3), *San Yin Jiao* (Sp 6), *Tai Xi* (Ki 3)

Key advice: This pattern is essentially another counterflow pattern. However, here the symptoms are a mixture of hot and cold, repletion and vacuity ones. This is a commonly seen pattern in Western patients.

Liver Blood, Kidney Yin Vacuity

Disease causes, disease mechanisms: This pattern may be due to congenital insufficiency or to overtaxation, prolonged disease, and aging, all of which consume and damage yin blood. Thus the various symptoms pertaining specifically to the liver are all those resulting from a lack of nourishment to the tissues associated with liver blood.

Main symptoms: Vexatious heat in the five hearts, insomnia, restless sleep, tidal fever, flushed cheeks in the afternoon, a dry mouth at night, night sweats, blurred vision or night blindness, dizziness, tremors and contraction of the sinews and muscles, numbness of the limbs, fragile nails, lateral costal pain, early menstruation, scanty menstruation, painful menstruation

Tongue & coating: A red tongue with scanty coating or a pale tongue with a red tip

Pulse image: A fine, wiry, perhaps even fast pulse

Treatment principles: Nourish the liver and supplement yin

Rx: *Qi Ju Di Huang Wan* (Lycium & Chrysanthemum Rehmannia Pills)

Ingredients:

Fructus Lycii Chinensis (*Gou Qi Zi*)
Flos Chrysanthemi Morifolii (*Ju Hua*)
prepared Radix Rehmanniae (*Shu Di Huang*)
Fructus Corni Officinalis (*Shan Zhu Yu*)
dry Radix Dioscoreae Oppositae (*Gan Shan Yao*)
Rhizoma Alismatis (*Ze Xie*)
Sclerotium Poriae Cocos (*Fu Ling*)
Cortex Radicis Moutan (*Mu Dan Pi*)

Additions & subtractions: For tremors and contraction of the sinews, add Fructus Chaenomelis Lagenariae (*Mu Gua*) and Radix Albus Paeoniae Lactiflorae (*Bai Shao*). For lateral costal distention and pain, add Fructus Meliae Toosendan (*Chuan Lian Zi*) and Tuber Curcumae (*Yu Jin*).

Acupuncture & moxibustion: *Gan Shu* (Bl 18), *Ge Shu* (Bl 17), *Qu Quan* (Liv 8), *San Yin Jiao* (Sp 6), *Guan Yuan* (CV 4)

Key advice: Many books title this pattern liver/kidney dual vacuity or liver/kidney yin vacuity. However, this obscures the fact that the liver vacuity is a blood vacuity.

Liver Blood, Kidney Yang Vacuity

Disease causes, disease mechanisms: Due to exhaustion of the *tian gui* perimeno-pausally, liver blood is typically deficient while kidney yin and yang are also vacuous and insufficient. Thus there is a combination of yin and blood vacuity symptoms mixed with yang vacuity symptoms seen below.

Main symptoms: Blurred vision or night blindness, dizziness, tremors and contractions of the sinews and muscles, numbness of the limbs, dizziness, tinnitus, fragile nails, lateral costal pain, scanty, light-colored menses, irregular menstruation, early menstruation, low back and knee soreness and weakness, loosening of the teeth, loss of hair, night sweats, hot flashes, cold feet, nocturia

Tongue & coating: A pale, swollen tongue with the indentations of the teeth on its edges and a red tip with a scanty coating

Pulse image: Floating, possibly surging pulses in the inch positions, wiry and fine images in the bar positions, and fine and floating in the left cubit

Treatment principles: Nourish the liver and supplement the kidneys, warm and strengthen kidney yang

Rx: *Er Xian Tang* (Two Immortals Decoction)

Ingredients:

Herba Epimedii (*Xian Ling Pi*)
Rhizoma Curculiginis Orchioidis (*Xian Mao*)
Radix Morindae Officinalis (*Ba Ji Tian*)
Radix Angelicae Sinensis (*Dang Gui*)
Cortex Phellodendri (*Huang Bai*)
Rhizoma Anemarrhenae (*Zhi Mu*)

Additions & subtractions: For night sweats, add Radix Ephedrae (*Ma Huang Gen*) and Fructus Levis Tritici Aestivi (*Fu Xiao Mai*). For fatigue, add Radix Panacis Ginseng (*Ren Shen*) and Radix Astragali Membranacei (*Huang Qi*). For insomnia, add Semen Zizyphi Spinosae (*Suan Zao Ren*) and Semen Biotae Orientalis (*Bai Zi Ren*). For hot flashes, add Concha Ostreae (*Mu Li*) and Concha Haliotidis (*Shi Jue Ming*). For low back pain, including that from osteoporosis, add Radix Dipsaci (*Xu Duan*) and Cortex Eucommiae Ulmoidis (*Du Zhong*). For spleen vacuity with loose stools and fatigue, add *Si Jun Zi Tang* (Four Gentlemen Decoction).

Acupuncture & moxibustion: *Gan Shu* (Bl 18), *Shen Shu* (Bl 23), *Ming Men* (GV 4), *Tai Chong* (Liv 3), *San Yin Jiao* (Sp 6), *Tai Xi* (Ki 3), *Guan Yuan* (CV 4)

Auxiliary points: For fatigue, add *Zu San Li* (St 36). For night sweats, add *Hou Xi* (SI 3). For palpitations and insomnia, add *Shen Men* (Ht 7) and *Nei Guan* (Per 6).

Key advice: This is one of the most common patterns among Western women beginning even as early as 35 years of age. It can be associated with luteal phase defect infertility, a progesterone deficiency, severe PMS, chronic breast disease, osteoporosis, and a host of menopausal complaints. Because there is heat above and cold below, symptoms of cold, such as cold feet, may be overlooked. The tongue may be reddish due to the counter-flowing vacuous yang qi and the pulse may be slightly rapid or at least not slow because of the vacuity heat. This pattern is very commonly complicated by both spleen qi vacuity and liver depression, qi stagnation since it typically evolves out of those two patterns.

Cold Stagnating in the Liver Vessels

Disease causes, disease mechanisms: This pattern is usually associated with vacuity cold. In this case, cold congeals the flow of qi and blood. Because there is no free flow, there is pain.

Main symptoms: *Shan* or lower abdominal pain that is sharp, localized, and aggravated by the local application of cold

Tongue & coating: A pale tongue, especially on the sides and root

Pulse image: A confined, tight pulse

Treatment principles: Warm the liver and scatter cold, rectify the qi and stop pain

Rx: *Nuan Gan Jian* (Warm the Liver Decoction)

Ingredients:

Radix Angelicae Sinensis (*Dang Gui*)
Fructus Lycii Chinensis (*Gou Qi Zi*)
Fructus Foeniculi Vulgaris (*Xiao Hui Xiang*)
Cortex Cinnamomi (*Rou Gui*)
Radix Linderae Strychnifoliae (*Wu Yao*)
Lignum Aquilariae Agallochae (*Chen Xiang*)
Sclerotium Poriae Cocos (*Fu Ling*)
uncooked Rhizoma Zingiberis (*Sheng Jiang*)

Additions & subtractions: For pain of the scrotum, add Semen Litchi Chinensis (*Li Zhi He*) and Semen Citri Reticulatae (*Ju He*). For severe pain in the lower abdomen, add Rhizoma Corydalis Yanhusuo (*Yan Hu Suo*) and Fructus Meliae Toosendan (*Chuan Lian Zi*).

Acupuncture & moxibustion: *Qi Chong* (St 30), *Tai Chong* (Liv 3), *Qu Quan* (Liv 8), *Qi Hai* (CV 6), *Zu San Li* (St 36), *Shen Que* (CV 8), and moxa over the affected area

Key advice: This pattern may be associated with testicular cancer. Therefore, the practitioner should palpate the testicles to see if there are any lumps or nodulations. If there are, the patient should be referred to a Western physician for further diagnosis.

The reason this pattern is called cold stagnating in the liver vessels and not the liver channel is that the cold is affecting the liver network channels that traverse the external genitalia. When this pattern occurs in a woman, causing painful menstruation and infertility, it is usually referred to as *bao han*, cold uterus.

Damp Heat Accumulating in the Liver & Gallbladder

Disease causes, disease mechanisms: This pattern is due to either invasion by damp heat evils from outside or overeating hot, acrid, peppery, greasy, fatty, thick-flavored foods, or drinking too much alcohol. This then causes heat in the liver and dampness in the spleen, which combine to form what has come to be called liver/-gallbladder damp heat.

Main symptoms: A bright yellow-colored body, face, and eyes, a bitter taste in the mouth, lateral costal distention and pain, nausea, vomiting, lack of appetite, aversion to fatty foods, alternating fever and chills

Tongue & coating: A slimy, yellow tongue coating

Pulse image: A slippery, rapid pulse

Treatment principles: Clear heat and disinhibit dampness, recede yellowing

Rx: *Yin Chen Hao Tang* (Artemisia Capillaris Decoction)

Ingredients:

Herba Artemisiae Capillaris (Yin Chen Hao)
Fructus Gardeniae Jasminoidis (Zhi Zi)
Radix Et Rhizoma Rhei (Da Huang)

Additions & subtractions: For high fever due to severe heat, add Radix Gentianae Scabrae (*Long Dan Cao*), Radix Isatidis Seu Baphicacanthi (*Ban Lan Gen*), and Radix Et Rhizoma Polygoni Cuspidati (*Hu Zhang*). For a bitter taste in the mouth, also add Gentiana. For serious cases of hepatitis with jaundice, spirit and orientation (*i.e.*, the emotions) befuddled and confused, and a yellow, slimy tongue coating, add Rhizoma Polygoni Cuspidati (*Hu Zhang*) and Rhizoma Acori Graminei (*Shi Chang Pu*). If there is delirium, add *An Gong Niu Huang Wan* (Quiet the Palace Bezoar Pills). For alternating fever and chills with a bitter taste in the mouth, add Radix Bupleuri (*Chai Hu*) and Radix Scutellariae Baicalensis (*Huang Qin*).

Acupuncture & moxibustion: *Qi Men* (Liv 14), *Yin Ling Quan* (Sp 9), *Zhi Gou* (TB 6), *Zu San Li* (St 36), *Tai Chong* (Liv 3), *Yang Gang* (Bl 48)

Key advice: It is interesting to note that the bitter taste in the mouth is due to heat forcing the bile out of the gallbladder.

Gallbladder Qi Vacuity

Disease causes, disease mechanisms: This pattern is mainly due to enduring stress causing liver depression and qi stagnation, which then transforms into heat plus spleen qi vacuity resulting in excessive phlegm. This spleen qi vacuity may be due to overeating sweet, greasy, fatty foods, overtaxation, or overthinking and worry, which may all damage the spleen. Liver depression also counterflows onto the stomach causing upward counterflow and depressive heat in that bowel as well.

Main symptoms: Irritability, anxiety, insomnia, excessive dreams, dizziness, vertigo, nausea, vomiting, excessive phlegm, chest oppression, palpitations

Tongue & coating: A slimy tongue coating

Pulse image: A wiry, slippery pulse

Treatment principles: Rectify the qi and transform phlegm, clear the gallbladder and harmonize the stomach

Rx: *Wen Dan Tang* (Warm the Gallbladder Decoction)

Ingredients:

Caulis Bambusae In Taeniis (*Zhu Ru*)
Fructus Immaturus Aurantii (*Zhi Shi*)
Rhizoma Pinelliae Ternatae (*Ban Xia*)

Pericarpium Citri Reticulatae (*Chen Pi*)
Sclerotium Poriae Cocos (*Fu Ling*)
Radix Glycyrrhizae (*Gan Cao*)
uncooked Rhizoma Zingiberis (*Sheng Jiang*)

Additions & subtractions: If there is qi vacuity, add Radix Panacis Ginseng (*Ren Shen*) and Fructus Zizyphi Jujubae (*Da Zao*). If there are a bitter taste in the mouth, a red tongue with a slimy, yellow coating, and a wiry, slippery, rapid pulse, add Rhizoma Coptidis Chinensis (*Huang Lian*). This then becomes *Huang Lian Wen Dan Tang* (Coptis Warm the Gallbladder Decoction). If there is severe vertigo, add Radix Albus Paeoniae Lactiflorae (*Bai Shao*), Heamatitum (*Dai Zhi She*), and Radix Scutellariae Baicalensis (*Huang Qin*). If there is insomnia, add Succinum (*Hu Po*), Semen Zizyphi Spinosae (*Suan Zao Ren*), and Concha Ostreae (*Mu Li*). If there is more severe insomnia, add Radix Panacis Ginseng (*Ren Shen*), Gypsum Fibrosum (*Shi Gao*), Tuber Ophiopogonis Japonicae (*Mai Dong*), Arillus Euphorbiae Longanae (*Long Yan Rou*), and Semen Zizyphi Spinosae (*Suan Zao Ren*).

Acupuncture & moxibustion: *Dan Shu* (Bl 19), *Shen Men* (Ht 7), *Xin Shu* (Bl 15), *Bai Hui* (GV 20)

Key advice: This formula's traditional name is misleading. In actuality, this pattern is a combination of disharmony between the gallbladder (*i.e.*, the liver), the stomach, and the heart and phlegm heat. Thus there are signs of qi depression, heat, phlegm, stomach disharmony, and a disquieted spirit. Important questions to ask in identifying this pattern are if the patient is easily startled, if they wake from sleep in a fright with possible palpitations, if they have excessive phlegm, and if they have a bitter taste in their mouth. Because of the relationships between the liver, spleen, stomach, and heart, there may also be signs and symptoms of spleen qi vacuity and heart blood vacuity.

Hyperactivity of Gallbladder Fire

Disease causes, disease mechanisms: This pattern may be due to anger, stress, and frustration, causing liver depression and qi stagnation plus overeating sweet, greasy, fatty, acrid, hot, peppery foods, and drinking too much alcohol. Thus liver depression transforms into heat, while at the same time there is depressive heat and loss of harmony in the stomach and spleen vacuity and dampness.

Main symptoms: Alternating fever and chills, chest and lateral costal region bitterness (*i.e.*, pain) and fullness, diminished intake of food and drink, heart vexation, nausea and vomiting, acid eructations, possible jaundice, a bitter or sour taste in the mouth, a dry throat, vertigo

Tongue & coating: A thin, white tongue coating

Pulse image: A wiry pulse

Treatment principles: Harmonize the liver and spleen and the spleen and stomach, resolve depression and clear heat

Rx: *Xiao Chai Hu Tang* (Minor Bupleurum Decoction)

Ingredients:

Radix Bupleuri (*Chai Hu*)
Radix Scutellariae Baicalensis (*Huang Qin*)
Radix Panacis Ginseng (*Ren Shen*)
Rhizoma Pinelliae Ternatae (*Ban Xia*)
Radix Glycyrrhizae (*Gan Cao*)
uncooked Rhizoma Zingiberis (*Sheng Jiang*)
Fructus Zizyphi Jujubae (*Da Zao*)

Additions & subtractions: If there is abdominal pain, subtract Scutellariae and add Radix Albus Paeoniae Lactiflorae (*Bai Shao*). Also for distension and pain, add Rhizoma Corydalis (*Yan Hu Suo*), Rhizoma Cyperi Rotundi (*Xiang Fu*), and Fructus Immaturus Aurantii (*Zhi Shi*). For sinusitis with a yellow nasal discharge due to gallbladder heat invading the brain, add Fructus Xanthii (*Cang Er Zi*), Herba Cum Radice Taraxaci Mongolici (*Pu Gong Ying*), and Herba Menthae Haplocalycis (*Bo He*). For muscle tension and chronic intestinal disorders with chilled extremities, add Ramulus Cinnamomi (*Gui Zhi*) and Radix Albus Paeoniae Lactiflorae (*Bai Shao*). This results in *Chai Hu Gui Zhi Tang* (Bupleurum & Cinnamon Twig Decoction). For nausea and vomiting add Caulis Bambusae In Taeniis (*Zhu Ru*).

Acupuncture & moxibustion: *Dan Shu* (Bl 19), *Yin Ling Quan* (Sp 9), *Qi Men* (Liv 14), *Xing Jian* (Liv 2), *Ri Yue* (GB 24), *Da Zhui* (GV 14)

Key advice: Although called hyperactivity of gallbladder fire, this is a complicated but commonly seen liver depression pattern in which there is depressive heat, spleen vacuity dampness, and loss of harmony of the stomach qi.

Heart & Small Intestine Patterns

Heart Qi Vacuity

Disease causes, disease mechanisms: Qi vacuity may be due to any of several causes: insufficient natural endowment, overtaxation, too much thinking and worry, enduring disease, aging, or blood loss.

Main symptoms: Palpitations and shortness of breath that are aggravated by exertion, anxiety, insomnia, poor memory, dizziness

Tongue & coating: A pale tongue with a thin, white coating

Pulse image: A fine, weak, regularly interrupted pulse

Treatment principles: Supplement the heart, nourish the blood, and quiet the spirit

Rx: *Yang Xin Tang* (Nourish the Heart Decoction)

Ingredients:

Radix Angelicae Sinensis (*Dang Gui*)
uncooked Radix Rehmanniae (*Sheng Di*)
prepared Radix Rehmanniae (*Shu Di*)
Sclerotium Pararadicis Poriae Cocos (*Fu Shen*)
Radix Panacis Ginseng (*Ren Shen*)
Tuber Ophiopogonis Japonicae (*Mai Men Dong*)
Semen Zizyphi Spinosae (*Suan Zao Ren*)
Semen Biotae Orientalis (*Bai Zi Ren*)
mix-fried Radix Glycyrrhizae (*Zhi Gan Cao*)
Fructus Schisandrae Chinensis (*Wu Wei Zi*)

Acupuncture & moxibustion: *Xin Shu* (Bl 15), *Shen Men* (Ht 7), *Gao Huang Shu* (Bl 43), *He Gu* (LI 4), *Zu San Li* (St 36), *Nei Gan* (Per 6)

Key advice: In actual fact, a heart qi vacuity by itself is seldom seen in clinical practice. Therefore, the majority of ingredients in this formula nourish the blood. The three ingredients that specifically supplement heart qi are the three ingredients of *Sheng Mai*

San (Engender the Pulse Powder): Ginseng, Ophiopogon, & Schizandra. This is because both the heart and lungs participate in the *zong* or gathering qi of the chest.

There are, in actuality, a couple of heart qi vacuity patterns described in the Chinese medical literature. One is heart qi not securing. This refers to the heart qi specifically not securing the heart spirit. This is characterized by heart spirit flightiness, essence spirit confusion, impaired memory, easy fright, spontaneous perspiration or sweating on movement.

The second subpattern of heart qi vacuity is heart qi vacuity inability to lie down. If the heart qi is insufficient, the heart spirit will not be tranquil and lying down to sleep at night will not be quiet. One is easily aroused from sleep and there are heart palpitations, lassitude of the spirit, lack of strength, a liking for warmth but aversion to chill, and a forceless or slow pulse. In order to boost the qi and nourish the heart, one can use either *Ren Shen Yang Rong Tang* (Ginseng Nourish the Constructive Decoction) or *Gui Pi Tang* (Restore the Spleen Decoction).

Ren Shen Yang Rong Tang: Radix Albus Paeoniae Lactiflorae (*Bai Shao*), Radix Angelicae Sinensis (*Dang Gui*), Pericarpium Citri Reticulatae (*Chen Pi*), Radix Astragali Membranacei (*Huang Qi*), Cortex Cinnamomi (*Rou Gui*), Radix Panacis Ginseng (*Ren Shen*), Rhizoma Atractylodis Macrocephalae (*Bai Zhu*), mix-fried Radix Glycyrrhizae (*Zhi Gan Cao*), prepared Radix Rehmanniae (*Shu Di*), Fructus Schizandrae Chinensis (*Wu Wei Zi*), Sclerotium Poriae Cocos (*Fu Ling*), Radix Polygalae Tenuifoliae (*Yuan Zhi*).

For the ingredients of *Gui Pi Tang*, see heart blood, spleen qi vacuity below.

Insufficiency of Heart Blood

Disease causes, disease mechanisms: Due to insufficient natural endowment, aging, enduring disease, or blood loss, there may be insufficient blood.

Main symptoms: Fright palpitations, restlessness, insomnia, excessive dreams, poor memory, suspiciousness, paranoia

Tongue & coating: A pale tongue with a thin, white coating

Pulse image: A fine pulse

Treatment principles: Supplement the heart and nourish blood

Rx: *Si Wu Tang* (Four Materials Decoction)

Ingredients:

Radix Angelicae Sinensis (*Dang Gui*)
Radix Ligustici Wallichii (*Chuan Xiong*)
Radix Albus Paeoniae Lactiflorae (*Bai Shao*)
prepared dry Radix Rehmanniae (*Shu Gan Di Huang*)

Additions & subtractions: For palpitations and dizziness, add Gelatinum Corii Asini (*E Jiao*) and Tuber Asparagi Cochinensis (*Tian Men Dong*). For insomnia, add Semen Biotae Orientalis (*Bai Zi Ren*) and Semen Zizyphi Spinosae (*Da Zao*).

Acupuncture & moxibustion: *San Yin Jiao* (Sp 6), *Yin Ling Quan* (Sp 9), *Xue Hai* (Sp 10), *Guan Yuan* (CV 4), *Qi Hai* (CV 6), *Ju Que* (CV 14)

Auxiliary points: For insomnia and disquieted spirit, add *Shen Men* (Ht 7).

Key advice: This is also an infrequently seen pattern in clinical practice. Its tongue and pulse signs are the same as those of liver blood insufficiency. However, the palpitations, insomnia, restlessness, paranoia, etc. all suggest that the spirit is not quiet because it is not being nourished.

Heart/Liver Blood Vacuity

Disease causes, disease mechanisms: Due to insufficient natural endowment, enduring diseases, aging, or blood loss, there may be insufficient blood to nourish the liver and heart. Thus the *hun,* or ethereal soul, and *shen,* or spirit, become restless. At the same time, insufficient yin and blood may give rise to symptoms of vacuity heat counterflowing upward and outward.

Main symptoms: Heart palpitations, night sweats, dizziness and vertigo, dry throat and mouth

Tongue & coating: A red tongue

Pulse image: A thready, rapid pulse

Treatment principles: Nourish the blood and quiet the spirit, clear heat and eliminate vexation

Rx: *Suan Zao Ren Tang* (Zizyphus Spinosa Decoction)

Ingredients:

Semen Zizyphi Spinosae (*Suan Zao Ren*)
Radix Glycyrrhizae (*Gan Cao*)
Rhizoma Anemarrhenae (*Zhi Mu*)
Sclerotium Poriae Cocos (*Fu Ling*)
Radix Ligustici Wallichii (*Chuan Xiong*)

Additions & subtractions: For vacuous heart and gallbladder qi with waking frightened in the middle of the night, a pale tongue and fine, wiry pulse, add Radix Codonopsis Pilosulae (*Dang Shen*) and Os Draconis (*Long Gu*). For palpitations, add Dens Draconis (*Long Chi*) and Concha Ostreae (*Mu Li*). For heart yin vacuity, add Tuber Ophiopogonis Japonicae (*Mai Dong*) and Semen Biotae Orientalis (*Bai Zi Ren*). For heart blood vacuity, add Arillus Euphoriae Longanae (*Long Yan Rou*), Radix Salviae Miltiorrhizae (*Dan Shen*), Cortex Albizziae Julibrissinis (*He Huan Pi*), and Caulis Polygoni Multiflori (*Ye Jiao Teng*).

Acupuncture & moxibustion: *Bai Hui* (GV 20), *Zu San Li* (St 36), *Shen Men* (Ht 7), *Xin Shu* (Bl 15), *Ge Shu* (Bl 17) *Gan Shu* (Bl 18)

Auxiliary points: For palpitations, add *Nei Guan* (Per 6).

Key advice: This pattern is a combination of liver and heart blood signs and symptoms plus vacuity heat symptoms counterflowing upward. It is a more commonly seen pattern than heart blood vacuity alone. It underscores the close relationship of liver blood to heart blood. The above formula is useful for treating night-crying and restlessness due to teething in babies.

Heart Blood & Yin Vacuity Inability to Lie Down

Disease causes, disease mechanisms: Due to internal damage by the seven emotions, heart blood and yin may be consumed. Thus the heart spirit is not nourished and loses its tranquility. This loss of tranquility is aggravated by vacuity heat disturbing the heart spirit as well.

Main symptoms: Vexatious heat in the five hearts, a dry mouth and tongue, fright when lying down to sleep at night

Tongue & coating: A red tongue with scant, dry coating

Pulse image: Fine and rapid

Treatment principles: Nourish the blood and enrich yin, clear heat and quiet the heart

Rx: *Huang Lian An Shen Wan* (Coptis Quiet the Spirit Pills) plus *Gui Shao Tian Di Jian* (Dang Gui, Peony, Asparagus & Rehmannia Decoction)

Ingredients:

Huang Lian An Shen Wan

Cinnabar (*Zhu Sha*)
Rhizoma Coptidis Chinensis (*Chuan Lian*)
uncooked Radix Rehmanniae (*Sheng Di*)
Radix Angelicae Sinensis (*Dang Gui*)

Gui Shao Tian Di Jian

Tuber Asparagi Cochinensis (*Tian Dong*)
prepared Radix Rehmanniae (*Shu Di*)
Radix Angelicae Sinensis (*Dang Gui*)
Radix Albus Paeoniae Lactiflorae (*Bai Shao*)

Acupuncture & moxibustion: *Shen Men* (Ht 7), *Nei Guan* (Per 6), *San Yin Jiao* (Sp 6), *Qu Quan* (Liv 8), *Xin Shu* (Bl 15), *Ge Shu* (Bl 17), *Gan Shu* (Bl 18)

Key advice: This pattern is essentially the same as heart/liver blood vacuity with vacuity heat described above. However, because its name is slightly different, we have included it for the sake of completeness in case a reader were to come across this pattern in the literature and not recognize it.

Cinnabar has been believed by Chinese to be relatively harmless when ingested because of poor intestinal absorption. However, experimentation with rats suggests that mercury poisoning can occur from internal administration of Cinnabar. Therefore, caution is advised when using this medicinal. It should not be used for any extensive period of time.

Heart/Spleen Dual Vacuity

Disease causes, disease mechanisms: The spleen is the postnatal or former heaven root of qi and blood transformation and engenderment. Excessive blood loss, faulty diet, overtaxation, or too much thinking and worry may all damage the spleen. Thus the spleen may fail to engender and transform qi and blood.

Main symptoms: 1) Heart palpitations, poor memory, insomnia, night sweats, vacuity heat (*i.e.*, feverishness), diminished appetite, bodily fatigue, a sallow yellow facial color; 2) hemafecia, uterine bleeding, early periods, excessive menstruation but pale colored blood, or dribbling and dripping that will not stop, or abnormal vaginal discharge

Tongue & coating: A pale, fat tongue with thin, white coating

Pulse image: A fine, relaxed or fine, weak pulse

Treatment principles: Boost the qi and supplement the blood, fortify the spleen and nourish the heart

Rx: *Gui Pi Tang* (Restore the Spleen Decoction)

Ingredients:

Radix Panacis Ginseng (*Ren Shen*)
Radix Astragali Membranacei (*Huang Qi*)
Rhizoma Atractylodis Macrocephalae (*Bai Zhu*)
Sclerotium Pararadicis Poriae Cocos (*Fu Shen*)
Arillus Euphoriae Longanae (*Long Yan Rou*)
Semen Zizyphi Spinosae (*Suan Zao Ren*)
Radix Auklandiae (*Mu Xiang*)
Radix Glycyrrhizae (*Gan Cao*)
Radix Angelicae Sinensis (*Dang Gui*)
Radix Polygalae Tenuifoliae (*Yuan Zhi*)

uncooked Rhizoma Zingiberis (*Sheng Jiang*)
Fructus Zizyphi Jujubae (*Da Zao*)

Additions & subtractions: For vacuous patients who cannot take large supplementing decoctions without experiencing abdominal distention and fullness, add Pericarpium Citri Reticulatae (*Chen Pi*) and Fructus Amomi (*Sha Ren*). For anemia, add Radix Ligustici Wallichii (*Chuan Xiong*) and Radix Albus Paeoniae Lactiflorae (*Bai Shao*). For edema, add Semen Coicis Lachryma-jobi (*Yi Ren*) and Rhizoma Alismatis (*Ze Xie*). For fallen qi, add Radix Bupleuri (*Chai Hu*) and Rhizoma Cimicifugae (*Sheng Ma*).

Acupuncture & moxibustion: *Xin Shu* (Bl 15), *Pi Shu* (Bl 20), *Zu San Li* (St 36), *Ge Shu* (Bl 17), *San Yin Jiao* (Sp 6), *Shen Men* (Ht 7)

Key advice: This is a commonly seen pattern in clinical practice. It is most frequently seen in women with a tendency to early or excessive menstruation or flooding and leaking.

Heart/Gallbladder Qi Vacuity

Disease causes, disease mechanisms: Dietary irregularity, enduring disease, overthinking, or overtaxation may all damage the spleen, in which case there is insufficient engenderment and transformation to nourish the heart and quiet the spirit. The spirit thus become restless, giving rise to symptoms such as susceptibility to fright and profuse dreaming.

Main symptoms: Timidity, susceptibility to fright, fatigue, heart palpitations, shortness of breath, reduced sleep, profuse dreaming

Tongue & coating: A pale tongue with thin fur

Pulse image: A weak pulse

Treatment principles: Supplement the qi, nourish the heart, and quiet the gallbladder

Rx: *Shi Wei Wen Dan Tang* (Ten Flavors Warm the Gallbladder Decoction)

Ingredients: Radix Panacis Ginseng (*Ren Shen*), 3g, mix-fried Radix Glycyrrhizae (*Zhi Gan Cao*), 3g, Sclerotium Poriae Cocos (*Fu Ling*), 9g, stir-fried Pericarpium Citri

Reticulatae (*Chen Pi*), 6g, lime-processed Rhizoma Pinelliae Ternatae (*Ban Xia*), 6g, Fructus Immaturus Aurantii (*Zhi Shi*), 6g, stir-fried Semen Zizyphi Spinosae (*Suan Zao Ren*), 9g, processed Radix Polygalae (*Yuan Zhi*), 9g, uncooked Fructus Schizandrae Chinensis (*Wu Wei Zi*), 9g, prepared Radix Rehmanniae (*Shu Di*), 6g

Acupuncture & moxibustion: *Shen Men* (Ht 7), *Qi Hai* (CV 6), *Xin Shu* (Bl 15), *Dan Shu* (Bl 19)

Key advice: This pattern is primarily a heart qi and blood vacuity pattern. However, because there is a pronounced element of timidity, and courage in Chinese medicine is believed to be a function of the gallbladder, gallbladder vacuity is also inferred. This pattern is similar to gallbladder qi vacuity discussed above except that there are no signs of heat. The key symptoms that distinguish this pattern are fear, fright, and waking up startled from sleep.

Heart Yang Vacuity

Disease causes, disease mechanisms: Overtaxation exhausts the heart qi and eventually, heart yang. It is also possible for heart yang to become vacuous and deficient due to enduring disease or debility due to aging.

Main symptoms: Heart palpitations, shortness of breath, cyanosis of the nails, chest pain, chilled limbs

Tongue & coating: A dark, purplish tongue

Pulse image: A regularly interrupted pulse

Treatment principles: Warm heart yang

Rx: *Shen Fu Tang* (Ginseng & Aconite Decoction)

Ingredients:

Radix Panacis Ginseng (*Ren Shen*)
Radix Lateralis Aconiti Carmichaeli Praeparata (*Fu Zi*)

Additions & subtractions: For stabbing chest pain, add Radix Salviae Miltiorrhizae (*Dan Shen*), Radix Rubrae Paeoniae Lactiflorae (*Chi Shao*), and Ramulus Cinnamomi (*Gui Zhi*). For fright palpitations, add Os Draconis (*Long Gu*) and Conch Ostreae (*Mu Li*).

Acupuncture & moxibustion: *Xin Shu* (Bl 15), *Shen Men* (Ht 7), *Shen Shu* (Bl 23), *Ming Men* (GV 4), *Tai Xi* (Ki 3), *Nei Guan* (Per 6)

Key advice: The above medicinal formula is not for chronic heart yang vacuity but for vacuity desertion. For a chronic heart yang vacuity, one might add Cortex Cinnamomi (*Rou Gui*) to the formula under heart qi vacuity. Because qi moves the blood and yang is only a lot of qi, this pattern is commonly complicated by blood stasis signs and symptoms, such as the cyanotic nails, dark, purplish nails, and stabbing chest pain.

Heart Blood Stasis

Disease causes, disease mechanisms: Due to enduring liver depression and qi stagnation, in turn due to anger and stress or to qi and blood vacuity due to disease or debility, blood flow in the heart may not be smooth and free-flowing. Thus stagnation may be retained, which then causes stasis and obstruction.

Main symptoms: Chest pain, dark lips or dark circles around the eyes, lancinating pain, possible nonstop hiccup lasting for many days, a choking sensation when drinking water, dry heaves, internal heat and oppression, possible heart palpitations, possible inability to sleep at night or one's sleep is not quiet, tension, agitation, easy anger, tidal fever

Tongue & coating: A dark red tongue, possible static patches or spots on the tongue

Pulse image: A choppy or wiry, tight pulse

Treatment principles: Quicken the blood and dispel stasis, move the qi and stop pain

Rx: *Xue Fu Zhu Yu Tang* (Blood Mansion Dispel Stasis Decoction)

Ingredients:

Semen Pruni Persicae (*Tao Ren*)
Flos Carthami Tinctorii (*Hong Hua*)
Radix Angelicae Sinensis (*Dang Gui*)

uncooked Radix Rehmanniae (*Sheng Di*)
Radix Ligustici Wallichii (*Chuan Xiong*)
Radix Rubrus Paeoniae Lactiflorae (*Chi Shao*)
Radix Achyranthis Bidentatae (*Niu Xi*)
Radix Platycodi Grandiflori (*Jie Geng*)
Radix Bupleuri (*Chai Hu*)
Fructus Aurantii (*Zhi Ke*)
Radix Glycyrrhizae (*Gan Cao*)

Additions & subtractions: For angina pectoris, increase the dosages of Carthamus and Ligusticum and add Radix Salviae Miltiorrhizae (*Dan Shen*).

Acupuncture & moxibustion: *Xin Bao Shu* (Bl 14), *Xin Shu* (Bl 15), *Ju Que* (CV 14), *Ge Shu* (Bl 17), *Xi Men* (Per 4)

Auxiliary points: In between acute attacks of pain, use *Xin Bao Shu* (Bl 14), *Xin Shu* (Bl 15), *Ge Shu (Bl 17)*, *Shan Zhong* (CV 17), *Nei Guan* (Per 6), *Xue Hai* (Sp 10)

Key advice: Patients with this pattern should be referred to a cardiologist for further tests and monitoring.

Phlegm Obstructing the Portals of the Heart

Disease causes, disease mechanisms: This pattern is mostly due to spleen vacuity and dampness engendering phlegm plus liver depression and qi stagnation, resulting in upward counterflow. This counterflow drafts the phlegm upward where it mists the portals of the heart, thus causing consciousness to be impaired. The spleen vacuity is due to overeating raw, chilled foods or sweet, fatty, thick-flavored foods, overthinking or too much worry, or overtaxation, which can all damage the spleen. The liver depression is due to anger and frustration causing the liver to lose control over orderly reaching.

Main symptoms: Emotional depression, withdrawal, muttering to oneself, staring at walls, sudden loss of consciousness of human affairs, no constancy in joy and anger, excessive, white phlegm, chest oppression, no thought for food or drink, the sound of phlegm rattling in the throat,

Tongue & coating: A thick, white, slimy tongue coating

Pulse image: A slippery, wiry, possibly bound pulse

Treatment principles: Rectify the qi and resolve depression, transform phlegm and open the portals

Rx: *Shun Qi Dao Tan Tang* (Normalize the Qi & Abduct Phlegm Decoction) plus *Kong Xian Dan* (Control Drool Elixir) with additions and subtractions

Ingredients:

Rhizoma Pinelliae Ternatae (*Ban Xia*)
Pericarpium Citri Reticulatae (*Chen Pi*)
bile[-processed] Rhizoma Arisaematis (*Dan Nan Xing*)
Sclerotium Poriae Cocos (*Fu Ling*)
Rhizoma Cyperi Rotundi (*Xiang Fu*)
Rhizoma Acori Graminei (*Shi Chang Pu*)
Radix Auklandiae (*Mu Xiang*)
Radix Euphorbiae Kansui (*Gan Sui*)
Radix Euphorbiae Seu Knoxiae (*Da Ji*)
Semen Sinapis Albae (*Bai Jie Zi*)

Acupuncture & moxibustion: *Jiu Wei* (CV 15), *Ju Que* (CV 14), *Shang Wan* (CV 13), *Zhong Wan* (CV 12), *Nei Guan* (Per 6), *Feng Long* (St 40)

Key advice: This pattern can be seen either as a liver pattern, in which case it is called phlegm qi depression and binding, or a heart pattern as above. It is due to liver depression, qi stagnation engendering phlegm, which then confounds the portals of the heart. It may also be called damp phlegm blocking the heart, phlegm turbidity confounding the pericardium, or phlegm confounding the portals of the heart. It is also similar to phlegm lodged in the chest and lateral costal regions.

If accompanied by chest pain or loss of consciousness, patients should be referred to a Western physician for diagnosis and monitoring, to be safe.

Phlegm Fire Harassing the Heart

Disease causes, disease mechanisms: This pattern is due to depressive heat stewing the juices and causing the engenderment of hot phlegm. This hot phlegm is drafted upward to the heart where the heat disturbs the heart spirit and the phlegm confounds the portals of the heart.

Main symptoms: Emotions tense and agitated, vexation and easy anger, both eyes looking angry, red face, red eyes, incessant talking, insomnia, a bitter taste in the mouth, excessive, yellow phlegm, chest oppression, constipation

Tongue & coating: A crimson red tongue with a thick, yellow, slimy tongue coating

Pulse image: A wiry, large, slippery, rapid, possibly urgent pulse

Treatment principles: Settle the heart and wash away phlegm, clear the liver and drain fire

Rx: *Sheng Tie Luo Yin* (Uncooked Iron Filings Drink)

Ingredients:

Frusta Ferri (*Sheng Tie Luo*)
bile[-processed] Rhizoma Arisaematis (*Dan Nan Xing*)
Bulbus Fritillariae (*Bei Mu*)
Radix Scrophulariae Ningpoensis (*Xuan Shen*)
Tuber Asparagi Cochinensis (*Tian Dong*)
Tuber Ophiopogonis Japonicae (*Mai Dong*)
Fructus Forsythiae Suspensae (*Lian Qiao*)
Ramulus Uncariae Cum Uncis (*Gou Teng*)
Radix Salviae Miltiorrhizae (*Dan Shen*)
Sclerotium Poriae Cocos (*Fu Ling*)
Sclerotium Pararadicis Poriae Cocos (*Fu Shen*)
Pericarpium Citri Reticulatae (*Chen Pi*)
Rhizoma Acori Graminei (*Shi (Chang Pu*)
Radix Polygalae Tenuifoliae (*Yuan Zhi*)
Cinnabar (*Zhu Sha*)

Additions & subtractions: If phlegm fire congests and is exuberant and the yellow, slimy tongue coating is severe, one can add *An Gong Niu Huang Wan* (Quiet the Palace Bezoar Pills) to clear the heart and open the portals.

Acupuncture & moxibustion: *Feng Fu* (GV 16), *Shen Zhu* (GV 12), *Da Zhui* (GV 14), *Ben Shen* (GB 13), *Lao Gong* (Per 8), *Feng Long* (St 40)

Key advice: This pattern may also be called phlegm fire blocking the heart.

Heart Yang Effulgence, Yin & Blood Vacuity

Disease causes, disease mechanisms: If, due to enduring stress and frustration, depressive heat counterflows upward to accumulate in the heart, it may eventually consume and damage yin and blood. In this case, yin blood will be unable to control and restrain heart yang, which then becomes effulgent and hyperactive.

Main symptoms: Heart vexation, spirit in chaos, insomnia, excessive dreams, fright palpitations, racing heart, if severe, a desire but inability to vomit, shortness of breath, forgetfulness

Tongue & coating: A red tongue or red-tipped, possibly ulcerated tongue

Pulse image: A rapid, thready pulse

Treatment principles: Settle the heart and quiet the spirit, drain fire and nourish yin

Rx: *Zhu Sha An Shen Wan* (Cinnabar Quiet the Spirit Pills)

Ingredients:

Cinnabar (*Zhu Sha*)
Rhizoma Coptidis Chinensis (*Huang Lian*)
Radix Angelicae Sinensis (*Dang Gui*)
uncooked Radix Rehmanniae (*Sheng Di*)
Radix Glycyrrhizae (*Gan Cao*)

Additions & subtractions: If heart fire is more prominent and there is more pronounced insomnia and vexation and agitation, add Plumula Nelumbinis Nuciferae (*Lian Zi Xin*) and Fructus Gardeniae Jasminoidis (*Zhi Zi*). Or specifically for insomnia, add Plumula Nelumbinis Nuciferae (*Lian Zi Xin*), Radix Polygalae Tenuifoliae (*Yuan Zhi*), and Sclerotium Pararadicis Poriae Cocos (*Fu Shen*). If the tip of the tongue is particularly red and dark or is ulcerated, accompanied by reddish-yellow, scanty urination, add Herba Lophatheri Gracilis (*Dan Zhu Ye*) and Medulla Junci Effusi (*Deng Xin Cao*).

Acupuncture & moxibustion: *Shen Men* (Ht 7), *Nei Guan* (Per 6), *Xin Shu* (Bl 15), *Shao Fu* (Ht 8), *Tai Xi* (Ki 3), *San Yin Jiao* (Sp 6)

Heart Fire Hyperactive Above

Disease causes, disease mechanisms: Fire in the heart develops from below. Either it is due to overeating sweet, greasy, fatty, acrid, hot, peppery foods and drinking alcohol, or it is due to overthinking, anger, stress, and frustration. In the first case, spleen damage leads to yin fire counterflowing upward, while in the second case, emotional depression and agitation cause ministerial fire to stir and counterflow up. Most cases in clinical practice are, in fact, due to a combination of these two factors.

Main symptoms: Heart palpitations, heart vexation, ulceration, swelling, and pain of the mouth and tongue, frequent, urgent urination

Tongue & coating: A red tongue

Pulse image: A rapid, slippery, possibly surging pulse

Treatment principles: Clear the heart and lead heat downward

Rx: *San Huang Xie Xin Tang* (Three Yellows Drain the Heart Decoction)

Ingredients:

Radix Scutellariae Baicalensis (*Huang Qin*)
Rhizoma Coptidis Chinensis (*Huang Lian*)
Radix Et Rhizoma Rhei (*Da Huang*)

Additions & subtractions: If heart heat is transferred to the small intestine and then to the bladder, add uncooked Radix Rehmannia (*Sheng Di*) and Caulis Akebiae (*Mu Tong*).

Acupuncture & moxibustion: *Tai Chong* (Liv 3), *Shen Men* (Ht 7), *Da Zhui* (GV 14), *He Gu* (LI 4), *Tai Xi* (Ki 3), *San Yin Jiao* (Sp 6), *Nei Guan* (Per 6), *Lao Gong* (Per 8)

Auxiliary points: If there is frequent, burning, urgent urination, add *Zhong Ji* (CV 3) and *Pang Guang Shu* (Bl 28).

Key advice: The difference between this pattern and the one above it is that, in this pattern, there are no signs of yin vacuity and there are *always* sores on the tip of the tongue. When this pattern is accompanied by urinary pain, frequency, and urgency, it is often referred to as heart and small intestine channel heat.

Patients with this pattern suffer concomitantly from polysystemic chronic candidiasis (PSCC). Therefore, they should be advised to stay away from foods that contain yeast, mold easily, or contain large amounts of sugar in any form. Such foods either damage the spleen or engender the accumulation of dampness. This then leads to yin fire flaring upward to disturb the heart with damp heat disturbing the bladder below.

Depressive Heat in the Heart Channel

Disease causes, disease mechanisms: This pattern is due to emotional stress and frustration, which results in depressive liver heat. This heat travels upward to accumulate in the heart. In addition, it is also due to undisciplined eating and drinking, such as overeating sweets and drinking too much alcohol. This results in a combination of spleen vacuity and stirring of ministerial fire with yin fire counterflowing upward to the heart. This pattern is called depressive heat because it is associated with a wiry pulse and emotional stress and is called heart channel because the skin rashes associated with this pattern often follow the course of the heart channel.

Main symptoms: Relatively small rashes that are red in color, burning hot, and itch. After scratching the skin with one's fingernails, raised rashes appear. This is accompanied by heart vexation, scanty sleep, and a dry mouth but no thirst.

Tongue & coating: A red tongue with a red tip and a thin, yellow coating

Pulse image: A fine and rapid or wiry, rapid pulse

Treatment principles: Cool the blood, clear the heart, and stop itching

Rx: *Liang Xue Xiao Feng San* (Cool the Blood & Disperse Wind Powder)

Ingredients:

uncooked Radix Rehmanniae (*Sheng Di*)
Radix Angelicae Sinensis (*Dang Gui*)
Herba Schizonepetae Tenuifoliae (*Jing Jie*)
Periostracum Cicadae (*Chan Tui*)
Radix Sophorae Flavescentis (*Ku Shen*)
Fructus Tribuli Terrestris (*Bai Ji Li*)
Rhizoma Anemarrhenae (*Zhi Mu*)
Gypsum Fibrosum (*Shi Gao*)
Radix Glycyrrhizae (*Gan Cao*)

Additions & subtractions: For more pronounced heat in the blood and for chronic cases, add Radix Rubrus Paeoniae Lactiflorae (*Chi Shao*) and Cortex Radicis Moutan (*Dan Pi*). For severe itching, add Bombyx Batryticatus (*Jiang Can*) and Lumbricus (*Di Long*). For trouble sleeping, add Concha Ostreae (*Mu Li*) and Caulis Polygoni Multiflori (*Ye Jiao Teng*).

Acupuncture & moxibustion: *Qu Chi* (LI 11), *He Gu* (LI 4), *Wei Zhong* (Bl 40), *Xue Hai* (Sp 10), *San Yin Jiao* (Sp 6), *Shao Fu* (Ht 8)

Key advice: This pattern, like other heart heat patterns, is often associated with an element of damp heat and spleen dampness. Commonly, such patients are prone to allergies and suffer from polysystemic chronic candidiasis (PSCC). Therefore, dietary therapy is as important as stress reduction in treating this kind of pattern. Patients with this pattern may, at other times, suffer from other of the heart heat/heart yang hyperactivity and/or from liver heat/liver yang hyperactivity patterns.

Heart Yin Vacuity

Disease causes, disease mechanisms: Due to insufficient natural endowment, aging, or overthinking and excessive worry and anxiety, yin and blood may be insufficient to control yang on the one hand and nourish the spirit on the other.

Main symptoms: Insomnia, excessive dreams, vexation and agitation, poor memory, tidal fever, night sweats, malar flushing, heart palpitations

Tongue & coating: A red tongue with scanty coating

Pulse image: A fine, rapid or floating, hooked pulse

Treatment principles: Supplement the heart and enrich yin, nourish the blood and quiet the spirit

Rx: *Bu Xin Dan* (Supplement the Heart Elixir)

Ingredients:

Radix Panacis Ginseng (*Ren Shen*)
Radix Scrophulariae Ningpoensis (*Xuan Shen*)
Radix Salviae Miltiorrhizae (*Dan Shen*)
Sclerotium Poriae Cocos (*Fu Ling*)
Fructus Schizandrae Chinensis (*Wu Wei Zi*)
Radix Polygalae Tenuifoliae (*Yuan Zhi*)
prepared Radix Rehmanniae (*Shu Di*)
Radix Platycodi Grandiflori (*Jie Geng*)
Radix Angelicae Sinensis (*Dang Gui*)
Tuber Asparagi Cochinensis (*Tian Men Dong*)
Tuber Ophiopogonis Japonicae (*Mai Men Dong*)
Semen Biotae Orientalis (*Bai Zi Ren*)
Fructus Zizyphi Jujubae (*Da Zao*)

Additions & subtractions: For dream-disturbed sleep and insomnia, add Caulis Polygoni Multiflori (*Ye Jiao Teng*) and Cortex Albizziae Julibrissinis (*He Huan Pi*).

Acupuncture & moxibustion: *Nei Guan* (Per 6), *Ju Que* (CV 14), *Shao Hai* (Ht 3), *Tai Xi* (Ki 3), *Fu Liu* (Ki 7), *Jin Men* (Bl 63)

Key advice: Although many textbooks list the pulse for this pattern as deep, fine, and rapid, often and especially in the inch positions, it is seemingly large, possibly slippery, but in that case, definitely floating. This adds up to the surging or hook-like pulse that is associated with the heart. It indicates that yin has lost control of yang, which is now counterflowing upward.

As the acupuncture formula above implies, although this pattern is called heart yin vacuity, there is kidney yin vacuity underneath. Therefore, in clinical practice, one may also give a combination of *Tian Wang Bu Xin Dan* (Heavenly Emperor Supplement the

Heart Elixir) and *Zhi Bai Di Huang Wan* (Anemarrhena & Phellodendron Rehmannia Pills).

Heart & Kidneys Not Interacting

Disease causes, disease mechanisms: If yin vacuity gets even worse, the heart and kidneys may no longer join or interact. Thus there are even more signs of heat above in conjunction with a disquieted spirit, while below there are signs of kidney vacuity weakness.

Main symptoms: Vexation and agitation, vexatious heat in the chest, restlessness, severe, continuous palpitations or racing heart, coolness of the lower limbs, great difficulty in falling asleep

Tongue & coating: A red tongue with a dry, yellow coating

Pulse image: A fine, rapid pulse or a surging pulse as described above

Treatment principles: Clear the heart and lead yang to move downward to its lower origin

Rx: *Jiao Tai Wan* (Grand Communication Pill)

Ingredients:

Rhizoma Coptidis (*Huang Lian*)
Cortex Cinnamomi (*Rou Gui*)

Acupuncture & moxibustion: *Tai Xi* (Ki 3), *Shen Men* (Ht 7), *Nei Guan* (Per 6), *San Yin Jiao* (Sp 6), *Xin Shu* (Bl 15), *Shen Shu* (Bl 23)

Key advice: This is a more extreme form of the above pattern. However, in this case, there is heat above but cold below. This is because yang has lost its root in its lower origin and is counterflowing upward. Whereas, in the previous case, there is kidney vacuity below, but it is yin vacuity without any signs of cold below.

Summerheat Entering the Heart Constructive (Aspect)

Disease causes, disease mechanisms: If summerheat invades the constructive aspect, the heart may be disturbed. This is because of the close relationship of the constructive to the blood and the blood to the heart.

Main symptoms: High fever that worsens at night, severe irritability, restlessness, disturbed sleep with possible delirium, cold limbs, deep, short breaths like in asthma, possible slight lockjaw

Tongue & coating: A crimson, dry tongue

Pulse image: A fine, rapid pulse

Treatment principles: Cool the constructive, clear the heart, and arouse the spirit

Rx: *Qing Ying Tang* (Clear the Constructive Decoction)

Ingredients:

Cornu Rhinocerotis (*Xi Jiao*)
Radix Scrophulariae Ningpoensis (*Xuan Shen*)
uncooked Radix Rehmanniae (*Sheng Di*)
Tuber Ophiopogonis Japonicae (*Mai Men Dong*)
Flos Lonicerae Japonicae (*Jin Yin Hua*)
Fructus Forsythiae Suspensae (*Lian Qiao*)
Rhizoma Coptidis Chinensis (*Huang Lian*)
Herba Lophatheri Gracilis (*Dan Zhu Ye*)
Radix Salviae Miltiorrhizae (*Dan Shen*)

Additions & subtractions: For severe depletion of yin fluids, add Radix Glehniae Littoralis (*Sha Shen*) and Fructus Lycii Chinensis (*Gou Qi Zi*). For tremors and spasms, add Ramulus Uncariae Cum Uncis (*Gou Teng*), Cornu Antelopis Saiga-tatarici (*Ling Yang Jiao*), and Lumbricus (*Di Long*).

Acupuncture & moxibustion: *Tai Chong* (Liv 3), *Wei Zhong* (Bl 40), *Ran Gu* (Ki 2), *Gao Huang Shu* (Bl 43), *Shen Men* (Ht 7), *Jia Che* (St 6), *Guan Chong* (TB 1), *Yin Xi* (Ht 6)

Key advice: This pattern is categorized according to defensive, qi, constructive, and blood pattern discrimination as a constructive aspect pattern.

Substitute Cornu Bubali (*Shui Niu* Jiao) for Cornu Rhinocerotis and Goat Horn (*Shan Yang Jiao*) for Cornu Antelopis Saiga-tatarici due to the fact that these animals are endangered because of their use in Chinese medicine.

Summerheat Damaging the Heart & Kidneys

Disease causes, disease mechanisms: Summerheat may damage both the heart, causing disquietude of the spirit, and the kidneys, causing damage to kidney yin. Damage to kidney yin may eventually reach or affect liver blood and yin, causing loss of nourishment of the sinews and hence numbness.

Symptoms: Irritability, a burning hot sensation in the head, continuous thirst, emaciation

Tongue & coating: A dry, thin, crimson tongue with a dry, yellow coating

Pulse image: A fine, rapid or vacuous, scallion-stalk pulse

Treatment principles: Nourish yin and clear summerheat

Rx: *Lian Mei Tang* (Coptis & Mume Decoction)

Ingredients:

Rhizoma Coptidis Chinensis (*Huang Lian*)
Fructus Pruni Mume (*Wu Mei*)
Tuber Ophiopogonis Japonicae (*Mai Men Dong*)
uncooked Radix Rehmanniae (*Sheng Di*)
Gelatinum Corii Asini (*E Jiao*)

Acupuncture & moxibustion: *Shao Chong* (Ht 9), *Guan Chong* (TB 1), *Jian Shi* (Per 5), *Shen Shu* (Bl 23), *Tai Xi* (Ki 3)

Key advice: According to triple burner pattern discrimination, this is a lower burner pattern. One could also classify this pattern as a disease cause (*bing yin*) pattern, in which case, the disease cause is summerheat.

Small Intestine Qi Pain

Disease causes, disease mechanisms: If undisciplined eating and drinking lead to food retention and depression, the qi may also become depressed and stagnant, thus resulting in lower abdominal pain.

Main symptoms: Cramping pain and distension in the lower abdomen, borborygmus, cramping pain of the testes and scrotum

Tongue & coating: A pale tongue with a white coating

Pulse image: A wiry pulse

Treatment principles: Move the qi and disperse accumulations

Rx: *Mu Xiang Shun Qi Wan* (Saussurea Normalize the Flow of Qi Pills)

Ingredients:

Radix Auklandiae (*Mu Xiang*)
Radix Atractylodis (*Cang Zhu*)
Massa Medica Fermentata (*Shen Qu*)
Radix Linderae Strychnifoliae (*Wu Yao*)
Sclerotium Poriae Cocos (*Fu Ling*)
Cortex Magnoliae Officinalis (*Hou Po*)
Pericarpium Citri Reticulatae (*Chen Pi*)
Rhizoma Cyperi Rotundi (*Xiang Fu*)
Rhizoma Pinelliae Ternatae (*Ban Xia*)
Radix Atractylodis Macrocephalae (*Bai Zhu*)
Pericarpium Citri Reticulatae Viride (*Qing Pi*)
Semen Raphani Sativi (*Lai Fu Zi*)
Fructus Aurantii (*Zhi Ke*)
Fructus Amomi (*Sha Ren*)

Acupuncture & moxibustion: *Zhong Wan* (CV 12), *Qi Hai* (CV 6), *Shang Ju Xu* (St 37), *Xia Ju Xu* (St 39), *Tian Shu* (St 25)

Key advice: Although this is called small intestine pain pattern, one can also see these symptoms as indicative of liver qi stagnation affecting the lower abdomen or a liver wood invading spleen earth pattern. Jeremy Ross says this pattern is the same as stagnation of cold in the liver channel. However, there do not have to be cold signs and symptoms in this pattern, whereas there must be such cold signs and symptoms in stagnation of cold in the liver channel.

Small Intestine Replete Fire

Disease causes, disease mechanisms: Due to a combination of extreme emotionality transforming into fire and usually some lack of discipline in eating and drinking, fire is engendered in the heart as well as dampness, which seeps below. This fire is transferred to the small intestine since fire is yang and the small intestine is the yang paired bowel to heart yin.

Main symptoms: Vexatious heat in the heart and chest, a red facial complexion, thirst with a desire for chilled drinks, reddish, astringent, inhibited urination, lower abdominal pain, possible sores in the mouth and on the tongue

Tongue & coating: A red tongue with sores on its tip

Pulse image: A rapid, slippery pulse

Treatment principles: Clear heat and enrich yin, disinhibit water and open strangury

Rx: *Dao Chi San* (Abduct the Red Powder)

Ingredients:

uncooked Radix Rehmanniae (*Sheng Di*)
Caulis Akebiae (*Mu Tong*)
uncooked Radix Glycyrrhizae (*Sheng Gan Cao Xiao*)
Folium Bambusae (*Zhu Ye*)

Additions & subtractions: For severe oral ulceration and sores on the tongue, add Rhizoma Coptidis Chinensis (*Huang Lian*). For hematuria, subtract Bamboo Leaves and add Herba Cephalanoplos (*Xiao Ji*) and Herba Ecliptae Prostratae (*Han Lian Cao*) or add Cephalanoplos and Rhizoma Imperatae Cylindricae (*Bai Mao Gen*). For severe urinary tract infection, add Herba Cephalanoplos (*Xiao Ji*), Fructus Gardeniae Jasminoidis (*Zhi Zi*), and Semen Plantaginis (*Che Qian Zi*).

Acupuncture & moxibustion: *Xiao Chang Shu* (Bl 27), *Zhong Ji* (CV 3), *Tong Li* (Ht 5), *Yin Ling Quan* (Sp 9), *Nei Ting* (St 44)

Key advice: There is little difference between this pattern and heart fire hyperactive above. However, in heart fire hyperactive above, the emphasis is on the oral ulceration and disturbed heart spirit. In this pattern, the emphasis is on the frequent, burning, painful urination. However, the sores on the tip of the tongue are the indication that this heat in the bladder has been passed there from the heart to the small intestine and only thence to the bladder since the small intestine and bladder are both *tai yang*.

Small Intestine Vacuity Cold

Disease causes, disease mechanisms: This pattern may be due to constitutional yang vacuity, enduring disease, or overeating raw, chilled foods.

Main symptoms: Aversion to cold, diarrhea, pain in the abdomen relieved by pressure and by warmth, stomachache, vomiting of clear fluid, borborygmus, loose stool, frequent urination

Tongue & coating: A white, slimy tongue coating

Pulse image: A thin and slow or thin and wiry pulse

Treatment principles: Warm the small intestine and disperse obstruction

Rx: *Wu Zhu Yu Tang* (Evodia Decoction)

Ingredients:

Fructus Evodiae Rutacarpae (*Wu Zhu Yu*)
uncooked Rhizoma Zingiberis (*Sheng Jiang*)
Radix Panacis Ginseng (*Ren Shen*)
Fructus Zizyphi Jujubae (*Da Zao*)

Additions & subtractions: For severe cold, add Pericarpium Zanthoxyli Bungeani (*Chuan Jiao*) and dry Rhizoma Zingiberis (*Gan Jiang*). For epigastric pain, add Radix Salviae Miltiorrhizae (*Dan Shen*) and Radix Saussureae Seu Vladimiriae (*Mu Xiang*). For *shan* due to cold, add Radix Lateralis Praeparatus Aconiti Carmichaeli (*Fu Zi*).

Acupuncture & moxibustion: *Tian Shu* (St 25), *Zu San Li* (St 36), *Xia Ju Xu* (St 39), *Guan Yuan* (CV 4)

Key advice: This pattern is very similar if not identical to spleen yang vacuity or central yang vacuity cold. The key difference is that, in this case, there is also excessive urination and, in TCM, the small intestine plays a role in the formation of urine.

Spleen & Stomach Patterns

Food Stagnation in the Stomach and Epigastrium

Disease causes, disease mechanisms: This pattern is commonly due to overeating and overdrinking either episodically or habitually.

Main symptoms: Stomach and epigastric distension and pain, bad breath, acid regurgitation, nausea, loss of appetite, loose stool or constipation, frequent, foul-smelling flatulence

Tongue & coating: A thick, slimy tongue coating

Pulse image: A slippery pulse

Treatment principles: Harmonize the stomach and disperse accumulations

Rx: *Bao He Wan* (Protect Harmony Pills)

Ingredients:

Massa Medica Fermentata (*Shen Qu*)
Fructus Crateaegi (*Shan Zha*)
Semen Raphani Sativi (*Lai Fu Zi*)
Pericarpium Citri Reticulatae (*Chen Pi*)
Rhizoma Pinelliae Ternatae (*Ban Xia*)
Sclerotium Poriae Cocos (*Fu Ling*)
Fructus Forsythiae Suspensae (*Lian Qiao*)

Additions & subtractions: If abdominal distention is severe, add Fructus Immaturus Aurantii (*Zhi Shi*) and Cortex Magnoliae Officinalis (*Hou Po*). For heat transformed from stagnation, add ginger(-processed) Rhizoma Coptidis Chinensis (*Huang Lian*). If there is constipation, add Radix Et Rhizoma Rhei (*Da Huang*).

Acupuncture & moxibustion: *Tian Shu* (St 25), *Zhong Wan* (CV 12), *Liang Men* (St 21), *Zu San Li* (St 36), *Nei Ting* (St 44)

Auxiliary points: If there is headache, add *He Gu* (LI 4). If there is burping and belching, add *Nei Guan* (Per 6). If there is transformative heat, add *Qu Chi* (LI 11).

Key advice: This pattern is very common in children due to their immature spleen and stomach function. Therefore, this formula can be given at the first sign of almost every common pediatric disease in infants and toddlers. The key symptom is bad breath.

Spleen Qi Vacuity

Disease causes, disease mechanisms: This pattern may be due to overtaxation, undisciplined eating and drinking, overeating raw, chilled foods, undereating, over-thinking and too much worry, and also to the erroneous or prolonged use of bitter, cold medicinals, all of which may damage the spleen.

Main symptoms: A somber white facial complexion, a faint, lethargic voice, diminished appetite, lack of strength of the four extremities, loose stools

Tongue & coating: A pale tongue with a slightly slimy, thin, white coating

Pulse image: A relaxed pulse

Treatment principles: Boost the qi and fortify the spleen

Rx: *Si Jun Zi Tang* (Four Gentlemen Decoction)

Ingredients:

Radix Panacis Ginseng (*Ren Shen*)
Rhizoma Atractylodis Macrocephalae (*Bai Zhu*)
Sclerotium Poriae Cocos (*Fu Ling*)
Radix Glycyrrhizae (*Gan Cao*)

Additions & subtractions: If there is more prominent phlegm dampness, add Rhizoma Pinelliae Ternatae (*Ban Xia*) and Pericarpium Citri Reticulatae (*Chen Pi*). This creates *Liu Jun Zi Tang* (Six Gentlemen Decoction). If simply more prominent dampness, add Rhizoma Atractylodis (*Cang Zhu*) and Semen Coicis Lachryma-jobi (*Yi Yi Ren*). If there is concomitant qi stagnation, add Fructus Amomi (*Sha Ren*) and Radix Saussureae Seu Vladmiriae (*Mu Xiang*). This then becomes *Xiang Sha Liu Jun Zi Tang* (Saussurea &

Amomum Six Gentlemen Decoction). Add Radix Scutellariae Baicalensis (*Huang Qin*) if there is concomitant stomach heat.

Acupuncture & moxibustion: *Pi Shu* (Sp 20), *Wei Shu* (Bl 21), *Zu San Li* (St 36), *Zhong Wan* (CV 12), *Tian Shu* (St 25)

Auxiliary points: Add *Shang Qiu* (Sp 5) for more pronounced dampness. Also add *Feng Long* (St 40) for phlegm dampness. Add *Liang Men* (St 21) and *He Gu* (LI 4) for food stagnation.

Key advice: Spleen vacuity most commonly complicates a number of other patterns in clinical practice. These include liver invading the spleen, spleen and kidney vacuity, stomach heat and spleen vacuity, and qi and blood dual vacuity. It is not very common to diagnose spleen vacuity all by itself in Western patients. On the other hand, due to faulty dietary practices and overwork, most Western patients' patterns are complicated by an element of spleen vacuity.

Spleen Vacuity, Excessive Drooling

Disease causes, disease mechanisms: If the spleen qi is insufficient, it may not be able to command the fluids and humors. These then accumulate and overflow in the form of excessive drooling in infants.

Main symptoms: Excessive, clear, watery drooling in infants, lassitude of the spirit, a sallow yellow facial complexion, a blue vein at *Shan Gen* (the root of the nose), possible abdominal distention and cramping (*i.e.*, colic), pumping of the legs against the abdomen, relief of discomfort after passing gas, cool hands and feet

Treatment principles: Supplement and boost the spleen qi

Rx: *Shen Ling Bai Zhu San* (Ginseng, Poria & Atractylodes Powder)

Ingredients:

Radix Panacis Ginseng (*Bai Zhu*)
Rhizoma Atractylodis Macrocephalae (*Bai Zhu*)
Sclerotium Poriae Cocos (*Fu Ling*)
mix-fried Radix Glycyrrhizae (*Zhi Gan Cao*)

Radix Dioscoreae Oppositae (*Shan Yao*)
Semen Nelumbinis Nuciferae (*Lian Zi*)
Semen Coicis Lachryma-jobi (*Yi Yi Ren*)
Fructus Amomi (*Sha Ren*)
Radix Platycodi Grandiflori (*Jie Geng*)

Key advice: This is a specifically pediatric pattern. The blue vein at *Shan Gen* and the cold hands and feet are important diagnostic signs. Most of these babies have colic.

Spleen Qi Downward Fall

Disease causes, disease mechanisms: Due to enduring spleen vacuity and possible prolonged standing or excessive fatigue during birthing, the spleen qi may not be able to restrain or hold in place the abdominal contents. This results in gastroptosis, chronic hemorrhoids, uterine prolapse, falling fetus, and habitual abortion.

Main symptoms: Fatigue, dizziness on standing, lack of strength, scanty appetite, possible loose stools, sagging and distention in the lower abdomen, distention after eating, prolapse of the rectum or uterus

Tongue & coating: A pale, enlarged tongue with a thin, white coating

Pulse image: A short pulse not reaching the inch position or a vacuous, rootless pulse in the right bar position

Treatment principles: Fortify the spleen and boost the qi

Rx: *Bu Zhong Yi Qi Tang*

Ingredients:

Radix Astragali Membranacei (*Huang Qi*)
Radix Panacis Ginseng (*Ren Shen*)
Rhizoma Atractylodis Macrocephalae (*Bai Zhu*)
Radix Angelicae Sinensis (*Dang Gui*)
Radix Bupleuri (*Chai Hu*)
Rhizoma Cimicifugae (*Sheng Ma*)
Pericarpium Citri Reticulatae (*Chen Pi*)
mix-fried Radix Glycyrrhizae (*Zhi Gan Cao*)

Additions & subtractions: To increase the lifting ability of this formula, add Fructus Aurantii (*Zhi Ke*). For abdominal pain, increase the dosage of mix-fried Licorice and add Radix Albus Paeoniae Lactiflorae (*Bai Shao*). For abdominal distention, add Fructus Immaturus Aurantii (*Zhi Shi*), Cortex Magnoliae Officinalis (*Hou Po*), Radix Auklandiae (*Mu Xiang*), and Fructus Amomi (*Sha Ren*). For diarrhea, add Radix Auklandiae (*Mu Xiang*). For habitual abortion, add Cortex Eucommiae Ulmoidis (*Du Zhong*) and Semen Cuscutae (*Tu Si Zi*). For abnormal vaginal discharge, add Cortex Phellodendri (*Huang Bai*) and Rhizoma Atractylodis (*Cang Zhu*).

Acupuncture & moxibustion: *Zu San Li* (St 36), *Qi Hai* (CV 6), *Bai Hui*(GV 20), *Pi Shu* (Bl 20), *Wei Shu* (Bl 21)

Key advice: This pattern is due to the spleen inability to restrain or hold the abdominal contents in place or to raise the clear yang. A good question to ask in regard to this pattern is whether one gets dizzy easily when standing up.

Spleen Not Restraining the Blood

Disease causes, disease mechanisms: This pattern may be due to overtaxation, aging, enduring disease, or overthinking and worry damaging the spleen, causing the qi to be too vacuous to restrain the blood within its vessels. It may also be seen in constitutionally obese patients with obvious phlegm dampness or rheum. However, even in that case, it is still due to spleen qi vacuity.

Main symptoms: Hemafecia, uterine bleeding, early periods, excessive menstruation but pale-colored, watery blood or dribbling and dripping that will not stop, or abnormal vaginal discharge

Tongue & coating: A pale, fat tongue with the teeth marks indented on its edge and a thin, white coating

Pulse image: A fine, weak, or faint pulse

Treatment principles: Boost the qi and supplement the blood, fortify the spleen and nourish the heart

Rx: *Gui Pi Tang* (Restore the Spleen Decoction)

Ingredients:

Radix Panacis Ginseng (*Ren Shen*)
Radix Astragali Membranacei (*Huang Qi*)
Rhizoma Atractylodis Macrocephalae (*Bai Zhu*)
Sclerotium Pararadicis Poriae Cocos (*Fu Shen*)
Arillus Euphoriae Longanae (*Long Yan Rou*)
Semen Zizyphi Spinosae (*Suan Zao Ren*)
Radix Auklandiae (*Mu Xiang*)
Radix Glycyrrhizae (*Gan Cao*)
Radix Angelicae Sinensis (*Dang Gui*)
Radix Polygalae Tenuifoliae (*Yuan Zhi*)
uncooked Rhizoma Zingiberis (*Sheng Jiang*)
Fructus Zizyphi Jujubae (*Da Zao*)

Additions & subtractions: For metrorrhagia due to the spleen failing to control the blood, subtract Saussurea and Polygala and add Fructus Corni Officinalis (*Shan Zhu Yu*). For prolonged uterine bleeding, add Gelatinum Corii Asini (*E Jiao*), Folium Artemisiae Argyii (*Ai Ye*), and Gelatinum Cornu Cervi (*Lu Jiao Jiao*). If complicated by blood stasis, add Flos Carthami Tinctorii (*Hong Hua*) and Cortex Radicis Moutan (*Dan Pi*). And if bleeding has gone on so long that there is loss of securing and astringing, add Fructus Corni Officinalis (*Shan Zhu Yu*) and Fructus Schizandrae Chinensis (*Wu Wei Zi*).

Acupuncture & moxibustion: *Zu San Li* (St 36), *San Yin Jiao* (Sp 6), *Pi Shu* (Bl 20), *Gao Huang Shu* (Bl 43), *Ge Shu* (Bl 17), *Guan Yuan* (CV 4)

Auxiliary points: For uterine bleeding, add *Yin Bai* (Sp 1). For dizziness due to excessive blood loss, add *Bai Hui* (GV 20).

Key advice: This pattern is commonly seen in clinical practice but mostly among women. When the above formula is used for the treatment of bleeding due to spleen qi vacuity, its effects are usually very good.

Spleen Vacuity, Heart Palpitations

Disease causes, disease mechanisms: This pattern is the sequela of an external invasion of cold evils in the *tai yang* aspect that has taken advantage of an internal vacuity. If such an invasion is not treated in time, this pattern may manifest after 2–3 days. Because the spleen qi and heart blood become even more vacuous and weak, this leads to the arising of heart palpitations.

Main symptoms: Heart palpitations with restlessness, lassitude of the spirit, shortness of breath, a low-grade fever, cold and sore extremities, a lusterless complexion, reduced appetite

Tongue & coating: A moist, white coating

Pulse image: A slow, weak pulse

Treatment principles: Supplement spleen, harmonize the qi and blood

Rx: *Xiao Jian Zhong Tang* (Minor Fortify the Middle Decoction)

Ingredients:

Maltose (*Yi Tang*)
Ramulus Cinnamomi (*Gui Zhi*)
Radix Paeoniae Lactiflorae (*Shao Yao*)
mix-fried Radix Glycyrrhizae (*Zhi Gan Cao*)
uncooked Rhizoma Zingiberis (*Sheng Jiang*)
Fructus Zizyphi Jujubae (*Da Zao*)

Additions & subtractions: For more severe cold, substitute cortex Cinnamomi (*Rou Gui*) for Ramulus Cinnamomi. If there are signs of simultaneous qi stagnation, such as a wiry pulse and abdominal pain, add Radix Auklandiae (*Mu Xiang*) and Endothelium Cornei Gigeriae Galli (*Ji Nei Jin*). If there is concomitant diarrhea, add Rhizoma Atractylodis Macrocephalae (*Bai Zhu*).

Acupuncture & moxibustion: *Tai Bai* (Sp 3), *Da Ling* (Per 7), *Gong Sun* (Sp 4), *Nei Guan* (Per 6)

Key advice: The slow pulse shows invasion by cold, while the weak pulse shows spleen vacuity. Although this pattern is a complication of heart blood, spleen qi vacuity, because there is the presence of evil cold, it is not treated with *Gui Pi Tang* (Restore the Spleen Decoction), nor is it listed under heart patterns.

Spleen Vacuity, Qi Stagnation

Disease causes, disease mechanisms: This pattern is the sequela of excessive sweating therapy used for a *tai yang* aspect external invasion. The massive sweating damages the spleen qi, which loses its control over transportation and transformation. Thus dampness accumulates and this dampness blocks the free flow of the qi. Because the qi does not flow freely and smoothly, but rather stagnates and accumulates as well, there is abdominal distention.

Main symptoms: Abdominal distension and fullness that are relieved by pressure and warmth, devitalized eating and drinking, fatigue, lack of strength

Tongue & coating: A pale tongue with a thin, white coating

Pulse image: A deep, slow pulse

Treatment principles: Warm the middle and supplement the spleen, loosen the center and disperse distention

Rx: *Hou Po Sheng Jiang Ban Xia Gan Cao Ren Shen Tang* (Magnolia, Ginger, Pinellia, Licorice & Ginseng Decoction)

Ingredients:

Cortex Magnolia Officinalis (*Hou Po*)
uncooked Rhizoma Zingiberis (*Sheng Jiang*)
Rhizoma Pinelliae Ternatae (*Ban Xia*)
Radix Glycyrrhizae (*Gan Cao*)
Radix Panacis Ginseng (*Ren Shen*)

Acupuncture & moxibustion: *Shang Wan* (CV 13), *Qi Hai* (CV 6), *Gong Sun* (Sp 4), *Huang Shu* (Ki 16)

Loss of Harmony between Spleen & Stomach

Disease causes, disease mechanisms: Due to constitutional vacuity, enduring disease, overtaxation, or lack of discipline, the spleen may be too weak to transport and transform food and drink. In this case, food and liquids may accumulate in the stomach. Thus there is a combination of spleen vacuity and food stagnation.

Main symptoms: Fatigue, scanty appetite, lack of strength, abdominal distention, loose stools, borborygmus, flatulence, distension and fullness in the epigastrium, bad breath, burping and belching, acid regurgitation, vomiting, diarrhea

Tongue & coating: A pale tongue with a thick, slimy coating

Pulse image: A slippery, relaxed pulse

Treatment principles: Supplement the qi and fortify the spleen, harmonize the stomach and disperse accumulation

Rx: *Xiang Sha Liu Jun Zi Tang* (Auklandia & Amomum Six Gentlemen Decoction)

Ingredients:

Radix Auklandiae (*Mu Xiang*)
Fructus Amomi (*Sha Ren*)
Radix Panacis Ginseng (*Ren Shen*)
Rhizoma Atractylodis Macrocephalae (*Bai Zhu*)
Sclerotium Poriae Cocos (*Fu Ling*)
mix-fried Radix Glycyrrhizae (*Zhi Gan Cao*)
Rhizoma Pinelliae Ternatae (*Ban Xia*)
Pericarpium Citri Reticulatae (*Chen Pi*)

Additions & subtractions: If there is indigestion, add Massa Medica Fermentata (*Shen Qu*), Endothelium Corneum Gigeriae Galli (*Ji Nei Jin*), Fructus Crataegi (*Shan Zha*), and Fructus Hordei Vulgaris (*Mai Ya*). If there is abdominal distention, add Semen Raphani Sativi (*Lai Fu Zi*) and Pericarpium Citri Reticulatae Viride (*Qing Pi*).

Acupuncture & moxibustion: *Zhong Wan* (CV 12), *Liang Men* (St 21), *Nei Guan* (Per 6), *Zu San Li* (St 36), *Nei Ting* (St 44), *Pi Shu* (Bl 20), *Wei Shu* (Bl 21)

Key advice: The additions given above are necessary if there is both spleen vacuity and food stagnation retained in the stomach.

Spleen Vacuity with Stomach Heat

Disease causes, disease mechanisms: Due to overeating acrid, hot, peppery foods, greasy, fatty, fried foods, and raw, chilled foods, there is heat in the stomach at the same time that there is vacuity and dampness in the spleen.

Main symptoms: Epigastric fullness and distention, possible nausea, vomiting, or acid regurgitation, borborygmus, diarrhea

Tongue & coating: A swollen tongue with the indentations of the teeth on its edges and a yellow, slimy coating

Pulse image: Wiry and rapid

Treatment principles: Fortify the spleen and harmonize the stomach, clear heat and transform dampness

Rx: _Ban Xia Xie Xin Tang_ (Pinelliae Drain the Heart Decoction)

Ingredients:

Rhizoma Pinelliae Ternatae (_Ban Xia_)
Rhizoma Coptidis Chinensis (_Huang Lian_)
Radix Scutellariae Baicalensis (_Huang Qin_)
dry Rhizoma Zingiberis (_Gan Jiang_)
Radix Panacis Ginseng (_Ren Shen_)
mix-fried Radix Glycyrrhizae (_Zhi Gan Cao_)
Fructus Zizyphi Jujubae (_Da Zao_)

Additions & subtractions: If there is more pronounced dampness, remove the dry Ginger and add uncooked Rhizoma Zingiberis (_Sheng Jiang_). If there is more serious qi vacuity, increase the dosage of mix-fried Licorice.

Acupuncture & moxibustion: _Zhong Wan_ (CV 12), _Tian Shu_ (St 25), _Zu San Li_ (St 36), _Nei Ting_ (St 44), _Pi Shu_ (Bl 20), _Wei Shu_ (Bl 21)

Key advice: This pattern is commonly seen in clinical practice, especially amongst Westerners. There is a combination of symptoms of both stomach heat and spleen vacuity. In subclinical cases, there may only be the pulse and tongue signs with a history of digestive complaints and a large appetite with a tendency to eat acrid foods, fatty foods, and raw, chilled foods.

Spleen Vacuity Reaching the Lungs

Disease causes, disease mechanisms: Due to constitutional spleen vacuity, overtaxation, undisciplined eating and drinking, enduring disease, or aging, spleen vacuity may eventually result in spleen/lung dual vacuity.

Main symptoms: Shortness of breath, cough on exertion or talking, panting and wheezing, expectoration of thin, white phlegm, spontaneous perspiration, fatigue, poor appetite, possible loose stools

Tongue & coating: A pale tongue with a thin, possibly slightly slimy, white coating

Pulse image: A faint or vacuous and large pulse

Treatment principles: Fortify the spleen and supplement the lungs

Rx: *Bu Fei Tang* (Supplement the Lungs Decoction)

Ingredients:

Radix Panacis Ginseng (*Ren Shen*)
Radis Astragali Membranacei (*Huang Qi*)
prepared Radix Rehmanniae (*Shu Di*)
Fructus Schisandrae Chinensis (*Wu Wei Zi*)
Radix Asteris Tatarici (*Zi Wan*)
Cortex Radicis Mori Albi (*Sang Bai Pi*)

Acupuncture & moxibustion: *Pi Shu* (Bl 20), *Fei Shu* (Bl 13), *Feng Long* (St 40), *Tai Yuan* (Lu 9), *Zu San Li* (St 36)

Key advice: The spleen is the latter heaven or postnatal root of qi and blood transformation and engenderment. Thus there are both spleen vacuity symptoms, such as fatigue, scanty appetite, and, commonly and especially in children with this pattern, loose stools, and lung vacuity symptoms, such as coughing and wheezing on exertion, coughing after talking, and spontaneous perspiration.

Spleen Yang Vacuity

Disease causes, disease mechanisms: Spleen yang vacuity may be due to enduring spleen qi vacuity evolving into spleen yang vacuity or severe damage to the spleen due to enduring disease, aging, or overeating raw, chilled foods.

Main symptoms: Fatigue, lack of appetite, lack of strength, loose stools, dull pain in the abdomen, edema, abdominal distention and fatigue after eating, a cold body with chilled extremities

Tongue & coating: A swollen, pale tongue with teeth prints on its border and a thin, white, slightly slimy coating

Pulse image: A deep and weak, faint, relaxed, or even slow pulse

Treatment principles: Supplement the qi and warm the spleen

Rx: *Fu Zi Li Zhong Wan* (Aconite Rectify the Middle Pills)

Ingredients:

Radix Lateralis Praeparatus Aconiti Carmichaeli (*Fu Zi*)
dry Rhizoma Zingiberis (*Gan Jiang*)
Radix Panacis Ginseng (*Ren Shen*)
Rhizoma Atractylodis Macrocephalae (*Bai Zhu*)
mix-fried Radix Glycyrrhizae (*Zhi Gan Cao*)

Acupuncture & moxibustion: *Pi Shu* (Bl 20), *Wei Shu* (Bl 21), *Zu San Li* (St 36), *Zhong Wan* (CV 12), *Qi Hai* (CV 6), *Tian Shu* (St 25)

Key advice: This pattern is not that commonly met in clinical practice in the West. In my experience, it is more common to find both spleen and kidney yang vacuity than spleen yang vacuity.

Spleen/Stomach Vacuity Cold

Disease causes, disease mechanisms: This is due to overeating raw, chilled foods, constitutional vacuity, and enduring disease.

Main symptoms: Dull pain in the epigastric or abdominal region that is relieved by pressure and warmth and aggravated by cold, vomiting of watery fluids, abdominal distension, fatigue, chilled limbs

Tongue & coating: A pale tongue

Pulse image: A deep, slow pulse

Treatment principles: Fortify the spleen and supplement the qi, warm the middle and scatter cold

Rx: *Huang Qi Jian Zhong Tang* (Astragalus Decoction to Construct the Middle)

Ingredients:

Radis Astragali Membranacei (*Huang Qi*)
Ramulus Cinnamomi Cassiae (*Gui Zhi*)
Radix Albus Paeoniae Lactiflorae (*Bai Shao*)
mix-fried Radix Glycyrrhizae (*Zhi Gan Cao*)
uncooked Rhizoma Zingiberis (*Sheng Jiang*)
Fructus Zizyphi Jujubae (*Da Zao*)
Maltose (*Yi Tang*)

Acupuncture & moxibustion: *Pi Shu* (Bl 20), *Wei Shu* (Bl 21), *Zu San Li* (St 36), *Zhong Wan* (CV 12), *Gong Sun* (Sp 4), *Nei Guan* (Per 6)

Key advice: This pattern is essentially the same as spleen yang vacuity. However, emphasizing the cold in the name of this pattern also emphasizes the dull pain in the abdomen. Cinnamon is not as hot as Aconite, but Peony helps to relieve tension and thus stop pain.

Spleen/Kidney Yang Vacuity

Disease causes, disease mechanisms: This pattern is mostly due to insufficient natural endowment, enduring disease, aging, and overtaxation.

Main symptoms: Abdominal pain that is aggravated by cold, polyuria, nocturia, low back and knee soreness and weakness, aching and heaviness of the extremities, fatigued spirit, generalized edema, loose stools, dizziness, a heavy sensation in the head, heart palpitations, coughing, vomiting

Tongue & coating: A pale or dark, swollen tongue with tooth marks and a white, slimy coating

Pulse image: A deep, fine, forceless pulse

Treatment principles: Fortify the spleen and strengthen the kidneys, supplement the qi and warm yang

Rx: *Zhen Wu Tang* (True Warrior Decoction)

Ingredients:

Radix Lateralis Praeparatus Aconiti Carmichaeli (*Fu Zi*)
Rhizoma Atractylodis Macrocephalae (*Bai Zhu*)
Sclerotium Poriae Cocos (*Fu Ling*)
uncooked Rhizoma Zingiberis (*Sheng Jiang*)
Radix Albus Paeoniae Lactiflorae (*Bai Shao*)

Additions & subtractions: If spleen yang vacuity is pronounced and accompanied by diarrhea, delete Peony and add dry Rhizoma Zingiberis (*Gan Jiang*). For spontaneous sweating that will not stop due to yang vacuity failing to secure the exterior, add Radix Panacis Ginseng (*Ren Shen*), Radix Astragali Membranacei (*Huang Qi*), and Fructus Schisandrae Chinensis (*Wu Wei Zi*).

Acupuncture & moxibustion: *Pi Shu* (Bl 20), *Shen Shu* (Bl 23), *Qi Hai* (CV 6), *Zu San Li* (St 36), *Zhong Wan* (CV 12), *Guan Yuan* (CV 4)

Key advice: In clinical practice, the combination of spleen and kidney yang vacuity is commonly seen in women in their late 30s, through their 40s, and into their 50s. In that case, there may be fatigue, loose stools, cold feet, nocturia, low back and knee soreness and weakness, and early menstruation, erratic menstruation, or flooding and leaking. In such cases, one should use a combination of *Bu Zhong Yi Qi Tang* (Supplement the Center & Boost the Qi Decoction) and *Er Xian Tang* (Two Immortals Decoction) with additions and subtractions. The above formula is best for digestive complaints and edema due to spleen/kidney yang vacuity.

Spleen Vacuity, Damp Encumbrance

Disease causes, disease mechanisms: Due to constitutional insufficiency, enduring disease, lack of discipline in eating and drinking, overtaxation, and too much thinking and worry, the spleen qi may be insufficient to transport and transform liquids. These then accumulate as water dampness. It is also possible for external damp to invade the body causing damage to the spleen.

Main symptoms: Edema, dizziness, headache, bodily fatigue, chest and epigastric fullness and oppression, nausea, vomiting, a slimy, sweet taste in the mouth, diarrhea possibly containing white mucus, urinary difficulty

Tongue & coating: A swollen, pale tongue with the marks of the teeth on its edges and a thin, slimy, white coating

Pulse image: A soggy, fine, wiry fine, or slippery, relaxed pulse

Treatment principles: Fortify the spleen and eliminate dampness

Rx: *Wei Ling San* (Stomach Poria Powder)

Ingredients:

Sclerotium Poriae Cocos (*Fu Ling*)
Sclerotium Polypori Umbellati (*Zhu Ling*)
Rhizoma Atractylodis Macrocephalae (*Bai Zhu*)
Rhizoma Alismatis (*Ze Xie*)
Ramulus Cinnamomi (*Gui Zhi*)
Rhizoma Atractylodis (*Cang Zhu*)
Cortex Magnoliae Officinalis (*Hou Po*)
Pericarpium Citri Reticulatae (*Chen Pi*)
Radix Glycyrrhizae (*Gan Cao*)
uncooked Rhizoma Zingiberis (*Sheng Jiang*)
Fructus Zizyphi Jujubae (*Da Zao*)

Acupuncture & moxibustion: *Pi Shu* (Bl 20), *Zu San Li* (St 36), *Shang Qiu* (Sp 5), *Shui Fen* (CV 9), *Zhong Wan* (CV 12), *Qi Hai* (CV 6)

Auxiliary points: If there are urinary difficulties, remove *Shang Qiu* and add *Yin Ling Quan* (Sp 9) and *Zhong Ji* (CV 3).

Key advice: In most Western patients, if there is spleen vacuity, there is usually some degree of evil dampness. Because spleen vacuity and damp encumberance complicate so many other patterns in clinical practice, the combinations that one should keep in mind for this condition are the two *zhu*, Rhizoma Atractylodis Macrocephalae (*Bai Zhu*) and Rhizoma Atractylodis (*Cang Zhu*); Rhizoma Atractylodis Macrocephalae (*Bai Zhu*) and Sclerotium Poriae Cocos (*Fu Ling*); and Rhizoma Atractylodis (*Cang Zhu*) and Semen Coicis Lachryma-jobi (*Yi Yi Ren*).

Spleen Dampness Attacking the Lungs

Disease causes, disease mechanisms: If dampness is engendered by the spleen due to loss of control over its functions of transportation and transformation, even though this dampness may have had its origin in the middle burner, it may accumulate above in the lungs and upper burner where it manifests as phlegm. Thus it is said, "The spleen is the source of phlegm formation but the lungs are where phlegm is stored."

Main symptoms: Excessive, white-colored phlegm that is easily spit out, chest and diaphragm glomus and oppression, nausea and vomiting, fatigue of the body and limbs, possible vertigo and palpitations, edema, loss of appetite

Tongue & coating: A white, moist tongue coating

Pulse image: A slippery pulse

Treatment principles: Dry dampness and transform phlegm, rectify the qi and harmonize the center

Rx: *Er Chen Tang* (Two Aged [Ingredients] Decoction)

Ingredients:

Rhizoma Pinelliae Ternatae (*Ban Xia*)
Pericarpium Citri Reticulatae (*Ju Pi*)
Sclerotium Poriae Cocos (*Bai Fu Ling*)
Radix Glycyrrhizae (*Gan Cao*)

uncooked Rhizoma Zingiberis (*Sheng Jiang*)
Fructus Pruni Mume (*Wu Mei*)

Additions & subtractions: For poor appetite and loose stools, subtract Mume and add Radix Panacis Ginseng (*Ren Shen*) and Rhizoma Atractylodis Macrocephalae (*Bai Zhu*), or combine *Er Chen Tang* with *Si Jun Zi Tang* (Four Gentleman Decoction). For ulcers and gastric distress, add Cortex Magnoliae Officinalis (*Hou Po*), Rhizoma Atractylodis (*Cang Zhu*), and Fructus Zizyphi Jujubae (*Da Zao*). For damp heat in the middle burner, add Herba Agastachis Seu Pogostemi (*Hou Xiang*), Rhizoma Coptidis Chinensis (*Huang Lian*), Cortex Magnoliae Officinalis (*Hou Po*), and Semen Coicis Lachryma-jobi (*Yi Yi Ren*).

Acupuncture & moxibustion: *Pi Shu* (Bl 20), *Fei Shu* (Bl 13), *Feng Long* (St 40), *Chi Ze* (Lu 5), *Tai Yuan* (Lu 9), *Zu San Li* (St 36)

Key advice: This pattern is a progression from the one above. If enduring, dampness will congeal to form phlegm, which is then typically stored in the lungs. Whenever there is spleen vacuity and dampness, proper diet is essential for a lasting cure. This pattern, coupled with counterflow qi/depressive heat *and* kidney vacuity is often the underlying composite pattern in cases of seasonal respiratory allergies.

Damp Heat Smoldering in the Spleen

Disease causes, disease mechanisms: Damp heat may invade externally and lodge in the spleen and stomach. There it hinders digestion and blocks the normal secretion of bile. However, due to the heat, the bile is forced out of the gallbladder to suffuse the skin yellow.

Main symptoms: Low-grade fever, epigastric fullness and oppression, abdominal distention, nausea, vomiting, fatigue, lack of strength, whole body, face, and eyes bright yellow, slight abdominal fullness, oral thirst, inhibited urination

Tongue & coating: A slimy, yellow tongue coating

Pulse image: A deep, rapid, slippery pulse

Treatment principles: Clear heat, disinhibit dampness, recede yellowing

Rx: *Yin Chen Hao Tang* (Artemisia Capillaris Decoction)

Ingredients:

Herba Artemisiae Capillaris (*Yin Chen Hao*)
Fructus Gardeniae Jasminoidis (*Zhi Zi*)
Radix Et Rhizoma Rhei (*Da Huang*)

Additions & subtractions: For high fever due to severe heat, add Radix Gentianae Scabrae (*Long Dan Cao*), Radix Isatidis Seu Baphicacanthi (*Ban Lan Gen*), and Radix Et Rhizoma Polygoni Cuspidati (*Hu Zhang*). For hypochondrial and lateral costal pain and abdominal fullness, add Tuber Curcumae (*Yu Jin*) and Fructus Immaturus Aurantii (*Zhi Shi*). For nausea, vomiting, and indigestion, add Caulis Bambusae In Taeniis (*Zhu Ru*) and Massa Medica Fermentata (*Shen Qu*).

Acupuncture & moxibustion: *Pi Shu* (Bl 20), *Yang Gang* (Bl 48), *Zhong Wan* (CV 12), *Zu San Li* (St 36), *Yin Ling Quan* (Sp 9), *Qu Chi* (Lu 11)

Spleen Heat, Excessive Drool

Disease causes, disease mechanisms: If wind heat evils congest in the spleen channel above, they may cause excessive drooling.

Main symptoms: Excessive drooling in infants, milk and food do not go down, plus other signs of heat as a red face when crying, hot hands and feet, reddish fingernails, red lips

Treatment principles: Clear the spleen and discharge heat

Rx: *Xie Huang San* (Drain the Yellow Powder)

Ingredients:

Gypsum Fibrosum (*Shi Gao*)
Fructus Gardeniae Jasminoidis (*Zhi Zi*)
Radix Ledebouriellae Sesloidis (*Fang Feng*)
Herba Agastachis Seu Pogostemi (*Huo Xiang*)
Radix Glycyrrhizae (*Gan Cao*)

Key advice: This is a specifically pediatric pattern.

Spleen Yin Vacuity

Disease causes, disease mechanisms: This pattern is usually the result of enduring disease where there is both spleen vacuity and stomach heat. This heat in the stomach is most commonly depressive heat due to liver depression. Eventually the heat in the stomach consumes and exhausts stomach yin. Thus there are symptoms of spleen vacuity and even spleen dampness at the same time as there is stomach yin vacuity and heat.

Main symptoms: Dry mouth, easily quenched thirst, low-grade fever, burning heat in the epigastrium, trouble digesting food that is eaten, easily full after eating a small amount, distention and fullness after eating, loss of taste, dry lips and possible sores in the mouth, loss of facial luster, wasting of the flesh and emaciation, alternating constipation and diarrhea, lack of strength in the limbs and body, vexatious heat in the hands and feet

Tongue & coating: A red tongue with a peeled center or scanty coating

Pulse image: A fine, rapid, forceless pulse

Treatment principles: Use sweet and bland to supplement the spleen

Rx: *Yi Pi Tang* (Boost the Spleen Decoction)

Ingredients:

Radix Pseudostellariae Heterophyllae (*Tai Zi Shen*)
Sclerotium Poriae Cocos (*Fu Ling*)
Rhizoma Atractylodis Macrocephalae (*Bai Zhu*)
Radix Platycodi Grandiflori (*Jie Geng*)
Radix Dioscoreae Oppositae (*Shan Yao*)
Semen Nelumbinis Nuciferae (*Lian Zi Rou*)
Semen Coicis Lachryma-jobi (*Yi Yi Ren*)
Semen Euryalis Ferocis (*Qian Shi*)
Semen Dolichoris Lablabis (*Bai Bian Dou*)
Herba Dendrobii (*Shi Hu*)
Fructus Germinatus Oryzae Sativae (*Gu Ya*)
mix-fried Radix Glycyrrhizae (*Zhi Gan Cao*)

Acupuncture & moxibustion: *San Yin Jiao* (Sp 6), *Pi Shu* (Bl 20), *Yin Ling Quan* (Sp 9)

Key advice: This pattern's description is based on an article by Steven Clavey, "Spleen and Stomach Yin Deficiency." It should be compared to stomach yin vacuity below.

Stomach Qi Counterflowing Upward

Disease causes, disease mechanisms: This is frequently caused by depressive heat accumulating in the liver in turn due to stress. Depressive qi counterflows to the stomach causing its qi to lose its harmony and also counterflow upward, while heat is transferred from the liver to the stomach.

Main symptoms: Burping and belching, hiccup, nausea and vomiting, dry heaves, difficulty swallowing, a choking sensation in the throat, vomiting in the evening what was eaten in the morning, vomiting in the morning what was eaten in the evening

Tongue & coating: A tender, red tongue

Pulse image: A thready, rapid or vacuous, rapid pulse

Treatment principles: Downbear counterflow and stop hiccup, boost the qi and clear heat

Rx: *Ju Pi Zhu Ru Tang* (Orange Peel & Caulis Bambusae Decoction)

Ingredients:

Pericarpium Citri Reticulatae (*Ju Pi*)
Caulis Bambusae In Taeniis (*Zhu Ru*)
Fructus Zizyphi Jujubae (*Da Zao*)
raw Rhizoma Zingiberis (*Sheng Jiang*)
Radix Glycyrrhizae (*Gan Cao*)
Radix Panacis Ginseng (*Ren Shen*)

Additions & subtractions: For concomitant phlegm, add Tuber Ophiopogonis Japonicae (*Mai Men Dong*) and Herba Dendrobii (*Shi Hu*). For vomiting or hiccup due to stomach yin vacuity and disharmony, add Sclerotium Poriae Cocos (*Fu Ling*), Rhizoma Pinelliae Ternatae (*Ban Xia*), Tuber Ophiopogonis Japonicae (*Mai Men Dong*), and Folium Eriobotryae Japonicae (*Pi Pa Ye*). This results in *Ji Sheng Ju Pi Zhu Ru Tang* (*Aiding Life* Orange Peel & Caulis Bambusae Decoction). For vomiting due to stomach heat, subtract Ginseng, Licorice, and Red Dates and add Calyx Khaki Diospyros (*Shi Di*). This results in *Xin Zhi Ju Pi Zhu Ru Tang* (Newly Processed Orange Peel and Caulis Bambusae Decoction).

Acupuncture & moxibustion: *Zhong Wan* (CV 12), *Nei Guan* (Per 6), *Zu San Li* (St 36), *Gong Sun* (Sp 4)

Key advice: Perhaps a more meaningful way of seeing this pattern is as liver invading the stomach with spleen vacuity and stomach counterflow plus the possibility of some depressive heat.

Stomach Fire Hyperactivity

Disease causes, disease mechanisms: This is due to overeating acrid, hot, peppery foods, greasy, fatty foods, fried and grilled foods, and drinking too much alcohol. Thus heat accumulates in the stomach and intestines. Because heat and fire are both yang in nature, this heat travels upward affecting the face and head.

Main symptoms: Bright red, swollen, painful gums, toothache, sores in the mouth, bad breath, a dry, thirsty mouth and desire for chilled drinks, possible red eyes, frontal headache, easy anger, heart vexation, reddish urine, constipation

Tongue & coating: A red tongue with scanty fluids but a thick, yellow coating

Pulse image: Surging and large or slippery and rapid

Treatment principles: Clear the stomach and drain fire

Rx: *Qing Wei San* (Clear the Stomach Powder)

Ingredients:

Rhizoma Coptidis Chinensis (*Huang Lian*)
Rhizoma Cimicifugae (*Sheng Ma*)
Cortex Radicis Moutan (*Dan Pi*)
uncooked Radix Rehmanniae (*Sheng Di*)
Radix Angelicae Sinensis (*Dang Gui*)

Additions & subtractions: If there is strong thirst for chilled drinks, remove Dang Gui and add Radix Scrophulariae Ningpoensis (*Xuan Shen*) and Radix Trichosanthis Kirlowii (*Tian Hua Fen*). If there is constipation, add Radix Et Rhizoma Rhei (*Da Huang*).

Acupuncture & moxibustion: *Nei Ting* (St 44), *He Gu* (LI 4), *Qu Chi* (LI 11), *Da Zhui* (GV 14)

Auxiliary points: If there are bleeding gums, add *Xue Hai* (Sp 10). If there is toothache, add local points on the *yang ming*, such as *Di Cang* (St 4), *Jia Che* (St 6), etc.

Key points: The formula that is commonly given for this pattern in Chinese textbooks is *Da Cheng Qi Tang* (Great Order the Qi Decoction). However, most Western patients are not robust enough for this formula.

This pattern may also be referred to as stomach fire attacking the lungs. In that case, there is cough with expectoration of phlegm and blood, fever, vexation and agitation, a dry mouth and lips, chest pain and oppression, bad breath, constipation, a red tongue with a dry, yellow coating, and rapid or surging and rapid pulse. The formula is the same as above.

Stomach Heat/Yin Vacuity

Disease causes, disease mechanisms: If stomach heat endures for a long time, it will eventually consume and damage kidney yin. Thus there are symptoms of stomach heat mixed with yin vacuity signs and symptoms.

Main symptoms: Toothache, loose teeth, bleeding gums, frontal headache, irritability, low-grade fever, a dry mouth and thirst with desire for chilled drinks

Tongue & coating: A dry, red tongue with a yellow coating

Pulse image: A floating, slippery, vacuous, large pulse

Treatment principles: Drain heat and nourish yin

Rx: *Yu Nu Jian* (Jade Woman Decoction)

Ingredients:

Gypsum Fibrosum (*Shi Gao*)
uncooked Radix Rehmanniae (*Sheng Di*)
Rhizoma Anemarrhenae (*Zhi Mu*)
Tuber Ophiopogonis Japonicae (*Mai Dong*)
Radix Achyranthis Bidentatae (*Niu Xi*)

Additions & subtractions: For severe yin vacuity, add Herba Ecliptae Prostratae (*Han Lian Cao*) and Fructus Ligustri Lucidi (*Nu Zhen Zi*). For bleeding gums, double the amount of Gypsum and Achyranthes and add Rhizoma Imperatae Cyclindricae (*Bai Mao Gen*) and Cortex Radicis Moutan (*Dan Pi*). If there is a dark, purple tongue with no coating, add Radix Glehniae Littoralis (*Sha Shen*) and Herba Dendrobii (*Shi Hu*). If there is profuse sweating and strong thirst, add Fructus Schizandrae Chinensis (*Wu Wei Zi*).

Acupuncture & moxibustion: *Tai Xi* (Ki 3), *San Yin Jiao* (Sp 6), *Nei Ting* (St 44), *He Gu* (LI 4), *Qu Chi* (LI 11), *Xue Hai* (Sp 10)

Key advice: This pattern is similar to the preceding one except that here there is also an element of yin vacuity. Thus the pulse is floating and large but vacuous and the tongue coating is yellow but not so thick.

Stomach Yin Vacuity with Damp Heat

Disease causes, disease mechanisms: Enduring dampness and heat in the liver and stomach may damage and consume stomach yin. In this case, heat will flare upward accompanied by symptoms of both dryness and dampness.

Main symptoms: Swollen gums, sores in the mouth and on the tongue, possible red, painful eyes, low-grade fever, constipation, abdominal distention, oral thirst but no great desire to drink, constant hunger but abdominal discomfort after eating, possible urinary strangury, possible yellowing of the skin and eyes

Tongue & coating: A red tongue with a scant, slimy, yellowish coating

Pulse image: A fine, rapid, slippery pulse

Treatment principles: Clear heat and eliminate dampness, nourish the stomach and rectify the qi

Rx: *Gan Lu Yin* (Sweet Dew Drink)

Ingredients:

uncooked Radix Rehmanniae (*Sheng Di*)
Tuber Ophiopogonis Japonicae (*Mai Dong*)
Tuber Asparagi Cochinensis (*Tian Dong*)
Herba Dendrobii (*Shi Hu*)
Herba Artemisiae Capillaris (*Yin Chen Hao*)
Radix Scutellariae Baicalensis (*Huang Qin*)
Folium Eriobotryae Japonicae (*Pi Pa Ye*)
Fructus Immaturus Aurantii (*Zhi Shi*)
Radix Glycyrrhizae (*Gan Cao*)

Acupuncture & moxibustion: *Nei Ting* (St 44), *San Yin Jiao* (Sp 6), *Zhong Wan* (CV 12), *Wei Shu* (Bl 21)

Auxiliary points: If there is urinary strangury, add *Yin Ling Quan* (Sp 9) and *Zhong Ji* (CV 3). If there is jaundice, add *Yang Ling Quan* (GB 34) and *Yang Gang* (Bl 48). If there are sores in the mouth, add *He Gu* (LI 4) and *Di Cang* (St 4).

Key advice: Patients with this pattern usually suffer from chronic candidiasis. Therefore, they should avoid sweets, foods made through fermentation, acrid, hot, peppery foods, and alcohol.

Stomach Yin Vacuity

Disease causes, disease mechanisms: This pattern is mostly seen in older patients where stomach yin has been consumed by the process of living. If complicated by heat, it may also be due to habitual overeating of acrid, hot, peppery foods, fried foods, and drinking alcohol.

Main symptoms: Dry lips and mouth, difficulty in swallowing, acid regurgitation, hiccup, vomiting, dry heaves, clamoring stomach, a burning feeling in the epigastrium, hunger but inability to eat much, constipation with dry stools

Tongue & coating: A red tongue with little coating or a glossy, mirror-like coating

Pulse image: A thready, rapid pulse

Treatment principles: Nourish stomach yin with sweet and cool, rectify the qi and harmonize the stomach

Rx: *Mai Men Dong Tang* (Ophiopogon Decoction)

Ingredients:

Tuber Ophiopogonis Japonicae (*Mai Men Dong*)
Radix Panacis Ginseng (*Ren Shen*)
Rhizoma Pinelliae Ternatae (*Ban Xia*)
Semen Oryzae Sativae (*Geng Mi*)
Fructus Ziziphi Jujubae (*Da Zao*)
Radix Glycyrrhizae (*Gan Cao*)

Additions & subtractions: For severe hiccups, add Calyx Khaki Diospyros (*Shi Di*) and Flos Caryophylli (*Ding Xiang*). For vomiting, add Rhizoma Coptidis (*Huang Lian*) and Caulis Bambusae In Taeniis (*Zhu Ru*). For constipation, add Radix Scrophulariae Ningpoensis (*Xuan Shen*) and raw Radix Rehmanniae (*Sheng Di Huang*).

Acupuncture & moxibustion: *Nei Ting* (St 44), *Zhong Wan* (CV 12), *Qi Hai* (CV 6), *San Yin Jiao* (Sp 6), *Nei Guan* (Per 6)

Key advice: According to Steven Clavey, one of the important factors in distinguishing spleen yin from stomach yin vacuity is duration of disease. Diseases of recent onset and short duration tend to exhibit the pattern of stomach yin vacuity, while old diseases of long duration tend to exhibit the pattern of spleen yin vacuity.

Stomach Blood Stasis

Disease causes, disease mechanisms: Due to enduring qi stagnation, the blood in the stomach may become static. In this case, there will be stomach pain.

Main symptoms: Stabbing, piercing pain in the epigastrium, abdominal distention, pain that refuses pressure, black stools like tar, a darkish face

Tongue & coating: A dark tongue with static spots or macules and a thin, yellow coating

Pulse image: Wiry and choppy

Treatment principles: Quicken the blood and transform stasis, open the network vessels and stop pain

Rx: *Shi Xiao San* (Losing a Smile Powder) plus *Dan Shen Yin* (Salvia Drink) with Rhubarb and Licorice

Ingredients:

Feces Trogopterori Seu Pteromi (*Wu Ling Zhi*)
Pollen Typhae (*Pu Huang*)
Radix Salviae Miltiorrhizae (*Dan Shen*)
Lignum Santali Albi (*Tan Xiang*)
Fructus Amomi (*Sha Ren*)
Radix Et Rhizoma Rhei (*Da Huang*)
Radix Glycyrrhizae (*Gan Cao*)

Acupuncture & moxibustion: *Zhong Wan* (CV 12), *Tian Shu* (St 25), *Ge Shu* (Bl 17), *Wei Shu* (Bl 21), *Da Chang Shu* (Bl 25), *Xue Hai* (Sp 6), *He Gu* (LI 4), *Zu San Li* (St 36)

Key advice: Patients with this pattern may have either bleeding ulcers or a digestive tract cancer. Therefore, such patients should be referred to a Western physician for diagnosis.

Lung & Large Intestine Patterns

Wind Cold Raiding the Lungs

Disease causes, disease mechanisms: This pattern is due to the external invasion of evil wind and cold. These enter the exterior where cold constricts the minute network vessels and wind obstructs the free flow of the defensive qi. Thus the lung qi diffusing and free flow is congested and blocked. The lung qi accumulates and counterflows upward, causing coughing and sneezing. This drafts with fluids, which counterflow as phlegm and runny nose. The fever is due to the congestion and accumulation of defensive qi in the exterior.

Main symptoms: Cough, a husky voice, rapid breathing, itchy throat, cough with thin, watery phlegm that is white in color, stuffed nose, runny nose, headache, soreness and aching of the body and limbs, aversion to cold, fever, no sweating

Tongue & coating: A thin, white coating

Pulse image: Floating and tight

Treatment principles: Course wind and scatter cold, diffuse the lungs and stop coughing

Rx: *Ma Huang Tang* (Ephedrae Decoction)

Ingredients:

Herba Ephedrae (*Ma Huang*)
Ramulus Cinnamomi (*Gui Zhi*)
Semen Pruni Armeniacae (*Xing Ren*)
mix-fried Radix Glycyrrhizae (*Zhi Gan Cao*)

Additions & subtractions: If there is external cold but internal heat, add Gypsum Fibrosum (*Shi Gao*). If there is simultaneous yang vacuity, add Radix Astragali Membranacei (*Huang Qi*). If there is sore throat, reduce the dosage of Cinnamon by half and add Radix Trichosanthis Kirlowii (*Tian Hua Fen*) and Rhizoma Belamcandae Chinensis (*She Gan*). If there is panting, chest oppression, and coughing with white, watery, thin phlegm, add Fructus Perillae Frutescentis (*Su Zi*) and Pericarpium Citri Reticulatae (*Chen Pi*).

Acupuncture & moxibustion: *Feng Men* (Bl 12), *Fei Shu* (Bl 13), *He Gu* (LI 4), *Lie Que* (Lu 7)

Auxiliary points: If there is copious phlegm, add *Feng Long* (St 40). If there is coughing and chest oppression, add *Shan Zhong* (CV 17).

Key advice: In this pattern, although there is fever, there is either no or only a slightly itchy sore throat. The patient should be put to bed and encouraged to sweat.

Wind Heat Attacking the Lungs

Disease causes, disease mechanisms: If the external evils of wind and heat invade the exterior, the wind will cause congestion of the lung qi's diffusion and downbearing. Thus the lung qi will accumulate and then counterflow upward. This results in coughing and sneezing. The heat will cause inflammation, such as a higher fever, slight or no aversion to cold, and thicker, yellowish phlegm.

Main symptoms: Cough, a rough, raspy voice, more serious sore throat, a dry throat, thick, sticky phlegm or thick, yellow phlegm, occasional sweating that does not relieve the fever, yellow mucus running from the nose, oral thirst

Tongue & coating: A thin, yellow coating

Pulse image: Floating and rapid or floating and slippery

Treatment principles: Course wind and clear heat, diffuse the lungs and transform phlegm

Rx: *Sang Ju Yin* (Morus & Chrysanthemum Drink)

Ingredients:

Folium Mori Albi (*Sang Ye*)
Flos Chrysanthemi Morifolii (*Jue Hua*)
Fructus Forsythiae Suspensae (*Lian Qiao*)

Herba Menthae Haplocalycis (*Bo He*)
Radix Platycodi Grandiflori (*Jie Geng*)
Semen Pruni Armeniacae (*Xing Ren*)
Rhizoma Phragmitis Communis (*Lu Gen*)
Radix Glycyrrhizae (*Gan Cao*)

Additions & subtractions: For qi aspect dryness, add Gypsum Fibrosum (*Shi Gao*) and Rhizoma Anemarrhenae (*Zhi Mu*). If there is constructive aspect heat with a dark red tongue, add Radix Scrophulariae Ningpoensis (*Xuan Shen*), Cornu Bubali (*Shui Nui Jiao*), and uncooked Radix Rehmanniae (*Sheng Di*). If there is heat entering the blood aspect, remove Phragmites and Mint and add Tuber Ophiopogonis Japonicae (*Mai Men Dong*), uncooked Radix Rehmanniae (*Sheng Di*), Rhizoma Polygonati Odorati (*Yu Zhu*), and Cortex Radicis Moutan (*Dan Pi*). For severe thirst, add Radix Trichosanthis Kirlowii (*Tian Hua Fen*). For sticky, yellow phlegm that is difficult to expectorate, add Pericarpium Trichosanthis Kirlowii (*Gua Lou Pi*) and Bulbus Fritillariae Thunbergii (*Zhe Bei Mu*). For sore throat, add Fructificatio Lasiosphaerae Seu Calvatiae (*Ma Bo*) and Fructus Arctii Lappae (*Niu Bang Zi*). For sore, swollen glands, add Radix Scrophulariae Ningpoensis (*Xuan Shen*), Spica Prunellae Vulgaris (*Xia Ku Cao*), and Bulbus Fritillariae Thunbergii (*Zhe Bei Mu*). And for wind heat affecting the eyes, add Fructus Tribuli Terrestris (*Bai Ji Li*), Semen Cassiae Torae (*Jue Ming Zi*), and Spica Prunellae Vulgaris (*Xia Ku Cao*).

Acupuncture & moxibustion: *Feng Men* (Bl 12), *Fei Shu* (Bl 13), *He Gu* (LI 4), *Qu Chi* (LI 11), *Chi Ze* (Lu 5)

Auxiliary points: For high fever, add *Da Zhui* (GV 14). For severe sore throat, bleed *Shao Shang* (Lu 11).

Key advice: Where the authors live, in Colorado, patients almost never present the pattern of wind cold raiding the lungs. Mostly they present with this pattern and/or the following one. This pattern's key distinguishing features are prominent sore throat, no body aches, and no pronounced aversion to cold.

Wind Dryness Damaging the Lungs

Disease causes, disease mechanisms: If the external evils of wind and dryness invade the exterior of the body, wind once again will congest and block the lung qi's diffusion and downbearing. Thus there is qi accumulation and counterflow leading to coughing and sneezing. Dryness damages lung yin and causes a dry cough and a dry, sore throat.

Main symptoms: Dry cough, itchy, dry, painful throat, dry lips and nose, no or scanty phlegm, which is thick and stringy and, which is not easy to expectorate, or phlegm within which there are threads of blood, a dry mouth, stuffed nose, headache, slight aversion to cold, generalized fever

Tongue & coating: A red tongue with a thin, white or thin, yellow coating and scanty fluids

Pulse image: Floating and rapid or small and rapid

Treatment principles: Course wind and clear the lungs, moisten dryness and stop coughing

Rx: *Sang Xing Tang* (Morus & Armeniaca Decoction)

Ingredients:

Folium Mori Albi (*Sang Ye*)
Fructus Gardeniae Jasminoidis (*Zhi Zi*)
Semen Praeparatus Sojae (*Dan Dou Chi*)
Semen Pruni Armeniacae (*Xing Ren*)
Bulbus Fritillariae Thunbergii (*Zhe Bei Mu*)
Radix Glehniae Littoralis (*Sha Shen*)
Cortex Fructi Pyri (*Li Pi*)

Additions & subtractions: If there is a dry, itchy throat, add Radix Scrophulariae Ningpoensis (*Xuan Shen*) and Fructus Arctii Lappae (*Niu Bang Zi*). If there is thick, yellow phlegm, add Fructus Trichosanthis Kirlowii (*Gua Lou*) and Fructus Aristolochiae (*Ma Dou Ling*).

Acupuncture & moxibustion: *Lie Que* (Lu 7), *He Gu* (LI 4), *Feng Men* (Bl 12), *Fei Shu* (Bl 13), *Nei Ting* (St 44), *San Yin Jiao* (Sp 6)

Key advice: The direction of needling *Lie Que* should be toward, the wrist.

Summerheat Damaging the Lung Network Vessels

Disease causes, disease mechanisms: Summerheat may damage the network vessels of the lungs, causing the blood to flow recklessly outside its pathways. This then results in hemoptysis and subcutaneous bleeding. Because the invading qi also obstructs the clearing and depurating of the lungs, there arise cough and rapid dyspneic breathing.

Main symptoms: High fever, thirst, blurred vision, dizziness, abrupt hemoptysis, subcutaneous hemorrhage, cough, rapid dyspneic breathing

Tongue & coating: A red tongue with a yellow coating

Pulse image: A rapid pulse

Treatment principles: Clear heat and resolve toxin, cool the blood and stop bleeding

Rx: *Xi Jiao Di Huang Tang* (Rhinoceros & Rehmannia Decoction) plus *Yin Qiao San* (Lonicera & Forsythia Powder)

Ingredients:

Xi Jiao Di Huang Tang:

Cornu Rhinocerotis (*Xi Jiao*)
uncooked Radix Rehmanniae (*Sheng Di*)
Radix Rubrus Paeoniae Lactiflorae (*Chi Shao*)
Cortex Radicis Moutan (*Mu Dan Pi*)

Yin Qiao San:

Fructus Forsythiae Suspensae (*Lian Qiao*)
Flos Lonicerae Japonicae (*Yin Hua*)
Radix Platycodi Grandiflori (*Jie Geng*)
Herba Menthae Haplocalycis (*Bo He*)
Folium Bambusae (*Zhu Ye*)
uncooked Radix Glycyrrhizae (*Gan Cao*)
Herba Seu Flos Schizonepetae Tenuifoliae (*Jing Jie Sui*)
Semen Praeparatus Sojae (*Dan Dou Chi*)
Fructus Arctii Lappae (*Niu Bang Zi*)
Rhizoma Phragmitis Communis (*Lu Gen*)

Acupuncture & moxibustion: *San Yin Jiao* (Sp 6), *Xue Hai* (Sp 10), *Ge Shu* (Bl 17), *Shen Dao* (GV 11), *Lie Que* (Lu 7), *Feng Men* (Bl 12), *Fei Shu* (Bl 13)

Key advice: Because Rhinoceros horn is from an endangered species, always substitute Cornu Bubali (*Shui Niu Jiao*), but in a higher dose.

Phlegm Heat Depressing the Lungs

Disease causes, disease mechanisms: Due to invasion of evil heat, phlegm is engendered, which then obstructs the flow of qi. The qi accumulates and then counterflows. It is also possible for accumulation of phlegm to transform heat. In either case, upward counterflow due to qi stagnation and accumulation in turn due to phlegm obstruction is aggravated or facilitated by the heat.

Main symptoms: Chest pain, cough with thick, yellow phlegm, vexation and agitation

Tongue & coating: A yellow, slimy tongue coating

Pulse image: A wiry, slippery, rapid pulse

Treatment principles: Broaden the chest and resolve depression, clear heat and transform phlegm

Rx: *Qing Qi Hua Tan Wan* (Clear the Qi & Transform Phlegm Pills)

Ingredients:

bile[-processed] Rhizoma Arisaematis (*Dan Nan Xing*)
Radix Scutellariae Baicalensis (*Huang Qin*)
Fructus Trichosanthis Kirlowii (*Gua Lou*)
Rhizoma Pinelliae Ternatae (*Ban Xia*)
Fructus Immaturus Aurantii (*Zhi Shi*)
Pericarpium Citri Reticulatae (*Chen Pi*)
Semen Pruni Armeniacae (*Xing Ren*)
Sclerotium Poriae Cocos (*Fu Ling*)

Additions & subtractions: For high fever, add Gypsum Fibrosum (*Shi Gao*) and Rhizoma Anemarrhenae (*Zhi Mu*). For excessive phlegm, add Herba Cum Radice

Houttuyniae Cordatae (*Yu Xing Cao*) and Radix Trichosanthis Kirlowii (*Tian Hua Fen*). And if there is very gummy phlegm, remove the Pinellia and add Semen Benincasae Hispidae (*Dong Gua Ren*).

Acupuncture & moxibustion: *Fei Shu* (Bl 13), *Ge Shu* (Bl 17), *Chi Ze* (Lu 5), *Feng Long* (St 40), *He Gu* (LI 4)

Auxiliary points: To help broaden or expand the chest, add *Shan Zhong* (CV 17).

Key advice: This is a commonly met pattern in patients with an acute respiratory tract infection that has endured for several days.

Lung Heat Smoldering & Exuberant

Disease causes, disease mechanisms: If evil heat in the lungs becomes exuberant, it may transform into fire, which may then damage the blood vessels and lead to coughing of blood or blood-streaked phlegm.

Main symptoms: Cough, panting and wheezing, expectoration of thick, purulent, yellow phlegm, possible blood-streaked phlegm, pain in the chest, and flaring of the nostrils

Tongue & coating: A red tongue with a thick, yellow coating

Pulse image: A slippery, rapid pulse

Treatment principles: Drain fire and clear the lungs

Rx: *Xie Bai San* (Drain the White Powder)

Ingredients:

Cortex Radicis Mori Albi (*Sang Bai Pi*)
Cortex Radicis Lycii Chinensis (*Di Gu Pi*)
mix-fried Radix Glycyrrhizae (*Zhi Gan Cao*)
Bulbus Fritillariae Thunbergii (*Zhe Bei Mu*)
Radix Platycodi Grandiflori (*Jie Geng*)
Semen Trichosanthis Kirlowii (*Gua Lou Ren*)
uncooked Rhizoma Zingiberis (*Sheng Jiang*)

Additions & subtractions: If there is excessive, yellow phlegm, add Herba Cum Radice Houttuyniae Cordatae (*Yu Xing Cao*). For constipation, add Radix Et Rhizoma Rhei (*Da Huang*). If there is bloody phlegm or hemoptysis, add Rhizoma Bletillae Striatae (*Bai Ji*) and Folium Eriobotryae Japonicae (*Pi Pa Ye*).

Acupuncture & moxibustion: *Fei Shu* (Bl 13), *Chi Ze* (Lu 5), *Tian Tu* (CV 22), *Qu Chi* (LI 11), *Nei Guan* (Per 6)

Auxiliary points: If there is excessive phlegm, add *Feng Long* (St 40). If there is coughing of blood or blood-streaked phlegm, add *Xue Hai* (Sp 10)

Key advice: The difference between this and the preceding pattern is that heat is worse and phlegm is relatively less. Further, fire has damaged the vessels and so there is bleeding of fresh, red blood, which is expectorated above.

Lung Heat Transmitted to the Large Intestine

Disease causes, disease mechanisms: Because the lungs and large intestine share an interior/exterior relationship, evil heat in the lungs may be transmitted to the large intestine.

Main symptoms: Fever, cough, diarrhea with yellow, foul-smelling stool, a burning sensation around the anus, but neither hardness nor pain in the abdomen

Tongue & coating: A deep red tongue with a yellow coating

Pulse image: A rapid pulse

Treatment principles: Clear heat and stop diarrhea with bitter, cold medicinals

Rx: *Ge Gen Huang Lian Huang Qin Tang* (Pueraria, Coptis & Scutellaria Decoction)

Ingredients:

Radix Puerariae (*Ge Gen*)
Radix Coptidis Chinensis (*Huang Lian*)
Radix Scutellariae Baicalensis (*Huang Qin*)
mix-fried Radix Glycyrrhizae Uralensis (*Zhi Gan Cao*)

Additions & subtractions: If there are prominent exterior symptoms, add Flos Chrysanthemi Morifolii (*Ju Hua*). If there is a high fever with bloody or pussy stools, add Radix Pulsatillae Chinensis (*Bai Tou Weng*) and Cortex Fraxini (*Qin Pi*). If there is dampness and heat as indicated by a slimy tongue coating and a slippery, rapid pulse, add Flos Lonicerae Japonicae (*Jin Yin Hua*) and Semen Plantaginis (*Che Qian Zi*).

Acupuncture & moxibustion: *Da Zhui* (GV 14), *Shi Xuan* (M-UE-1-5), *He Gu* (LI 4), *Li Dui* (St 45), *Feng Chi* (GB 20), *Feng Men* (Bl 12), *Yu Ji* (Lu 10)

Damp Heat Smoldering in the Lungs

Disease causes, disease mechanisms: Damp heat smolders in the lungs, damaging the vessels. This results in bleeding and the formation of thick, purulent, yellow phlegm.

Main symptoms: Cough, wheezing, expectoration of excessive, thick, purulent yellowish phlegm, possible bloody, foul-smelling pus, relatively mild chest pain, low-grade fever, epigastric and diaphragmatic distention and oppression

Tongue & coating: A red, swollen tongue with a slimy, yellow coating

Pulse image: A slippery, rapid pulse

Treatment principles: Clear heat from the lungs and eliminate dampness, dispel stasis and discharge pus

Rx: *Qian Jin Wei Jing Tang* (*Thousand [Pieces of] Gold* Phragmites Decoction)

Ingredients:

Rhizoma Phragmitis Communis (*Wei Jing*)
Semen Coicis Lachryma-jobi (*Yi Yi Ren*)
Semen Benincasae Hispidae (*Dong Gua Ren*)
Semen Persicae (*Tao Ren*)

Additions & subtractions: If there is severe heat in the lungs, add Flos Lonicerae Japonicae (*Yin Hua*) and Herba Cum Radice Houttuyniae Cordatae (*Yu Xing Cao*). If the phlegm is very pussy, add Radix Platycodi Grandiflori (*Jie Geng*), Bulbus Fritillariae

Cirrhosae (*Chuan Bei Mu*), and Radix Glycyrrhizae (*Gan Cao*). If there is excessive phlegm, add Semen Descurainiae Seu Lepidii (*Ting Li Zi*).

Acupuncture & moxibustion: *Qu Chi* (LI 11), *Da Zhui* (GV 14), *Fei Shu* (Bl 13), *Ge Shu* (Bl 17), *Chi Ze* (Lu 5), *Nei Guan* (Per 6)

Key advice: This pattern describes abscess of the lungs. Damp heat might also be described as heat toxins. In addition to the damp heat, there is also an element of blood stasis due to obstruction by the dampness and heat.

Phlegm Turbidity Obstructing the Lungs

Disease causes, disease mechanisms: If, due to faulty diet or constitutional insufficiency, the spleen is vacuous and weak, spleen dampness may engender phlegm and this phlegm may flood the lungs above. This then congests and blocks the lung qi, which then accumulates and counterflows as coughing and panting.

Main symptoms: Coughing, excessive phlegm, the sound of the cough heavy and turbid, coughing because of phlegm, coughing levelled after the phlegm is discharged, thick, sticky phlegm or thick phlegm in the shape of lumps, white in color or grayish, coughing with excessive phlegm, worse after meals, worse after eating sweet, oily, slimy foods, chest oppression, epigastric glomus, nausea, bodily fatigue, occasional loose stools

Tongue & coating: A white, thick, slimy tongue coating

Pulse image: Soggy and slippery

Treatment principles: Fortify the spleen and dry dampness, transform phlegm and stop coughing

Rx: *Er Chen Tang* (Two Aged [Ingredients] Decoction plus *San Zi Yang Qin Tang* (Three Seeds Nourish [One's] Parents Decoction)

Ingredients:

Pericarpium Citri Reticulatae (*Chen Pi*)
Rhizoma Pinelliae Ternatae (*Ban Xia*)
Sclerotium Poriae Cocos (*Fu Ling*)

Radix Glycyrrhizae (*Gan Cao*)
Semen Sinapis Albae (*Bai Jie Zi*)
Fructus Perillae Frutescentis (*Su Zi*)
Semen Raphani Sativae (*Lai Fu Zi*)

Additions & subtractions: If cold phlegm is relatively heavy, the phlegm is sticky and white like glue, and there is fear of chill, add dry Rhizoma Zingiberis (*Gan Jiang*) and Herba Cum Radice Asari Sieboldi (*Xi Xin*). If there is enduring disease and spleen vacuity with fatigued spirit, add Radix Codonopsis Pilosulae (*Dang Shen*), Rhizoma Atractylodis Macrocephalae (*Bai Zhu*), and mix-fried Radix Glycyrrhizae (*Zhi Gan Cao*). Or one may add Rhizoma Atractylodis (*Cang Zhu*) and Cortex Magnoliae Officinalis (*Hou Po*) simply to increase the power of drying dampness and rectifying the spleen.

Acupuncture & moxibustion: *Fei Shu* (Bl 13), *Pi Shu* (Bl 20), *Shan Zhong* (CV 17), *Zu San Li* (St 36), *Feng Long* (St 40)

Key advice: After the coughing is arrested and the phlegm is eliminated, continue giving *Liu Jun Zi Tang* (Six Gentlemen Decoction) in order to secure the treatment effect.

Lung Qi Vacuity

Disease causes, disease mechanisms: This pattern is mostly due to enduring disease consuming the righteous qi of the lungs.

Main symptoms: Cough and panting worsened by exertion or speaking, shortness of breath, spontaneous sweating

Tongue & coating: A pale tongue with a thin, white coating

Pulse image: A faint or large, vacuous pulse

Treatment principles: Supplement the lungs and boost the qi

Rx: *Bu Fei Tang* (Tonify the Lungs Decoction)

Ingredients:

Radix Panacis Ginseng (*Ren Shen*)
Radix Astragali Membranacei (*Huang Qi*)

prepared Radix Rehmanniae (*Shu Di Huang*)
Fructus Schisandrae Chinensis (*Wu Wei Zi*)
Radix Asteris Tatarici (*Zi Wan*)
Cortex Radicis Mori Albi (*Sang Bai Pi*)

Acupuncture & moxibustion: *Zhong Fu* (Lu 1), *Fei Shu* (Bl 13), *Tai Yuan* (Lu 9), *Shan Zhong* (CV 17), *Zu San Li* (St 36)

Key advice: This condition is aggravated by anything that weakens either the spleen or the kidneys and in particular, overtaxation. Therefore, rest is crucial to the cure of this condition, as little talking as possible, and a clear, bland diet that is easy to digest and fortifies the spleen.

Lung/Spleen Qi Vacuity

Disease causes, disease mechanisms: Enduring, recurrent coughing due to lung qi vacuity eventually weakens the spleen as well.

Main symptoms: Cough, shortness of breath, clear, watery phlegm, a somber white facial complexion, spontaneous sweating, fear of wind, scanty appetite, torpid intake, loose stools, superficial edema of the face and four limbs

Tongue & coating: A pale tongue with the indentations of the teeth on its edges and a white coating

Pulse image: Soggy and weak

Treatment principles: Fortify the spleen and boost the qi, supplement earth to engender metal

Rx: *Liu Jun Zi Tang*

Ingredients:

Radix Panacis Ginseng (*Ren Shen*)
Rhizoma Atractylodis Macrocephalae (*Bai Zhu*)
Sclerotium Poriae Cocos (*Fu Ling*)
Rhizoma Pinelliae Ternatae (*Ban Xia*)

Pericarpium Citri Reticulatae (*Chen Pi*)
mix-fried Radix Glycyrrhizae (*Zhi Gan Cao*)

Acupuncture & moxibustion: *Fei Shu* (Bl 13), *Pi Shu* (Bl 20), *Wei Shu* (Bl 21), *Tai Yuan* (Lu 9), *Zu San Li* (St 36)

Key advice: Just as with phlegm turbidity obstructing the lungs, this pattern involves both the lungs and the spleen and, in particular, the spleen's ability to transport and transform liquids. However, phlegm turbidity is a replete pattern, whereas this is a vacuity pattern. Therefore, the pulse is soggy and weak as opposed to soggy and slippery.

Cold Rheum Deep-lying in the Lungs

Disease causes, disease mechanisms: This pattern is due to enduring disease eventually affecting the spleen yang or is seen in patients with spleen yang vacuity due to old age. Thus yin is exuberant and yang is debilitated and cold rheum is engendered internally. This then floods upward to hide in the lungs, disturbing the lungs' diffusion and downbearing.

Main symptoms: Cough with excessive phlegm that is thin, watery, and white, chest oppression, rapid breathing, if severe, panting and coughing which is worse in the fall and winter

Tongue & coating: A white, slimy or moist, glossy tongue coating

Pulse image: A vacuous or deep, fine pulse

Treatment principles: Warm and transform cold rheum

Rx: *Ling Gan Wu Wei Jiang Xin Tang* (Poria, Licorice, Schizandra, Ginger & Asarum Decoction)

Ingredients:

Sclerotium Poriae Cocos (*Fu Ling*)
Radix Glycyrrhizae (*Gan Cao*)
dry Rhizoma Zingiberis (*Gan Jiang*)
Herba Cum Radice Asari Sieboldi (*Xi Xin*)

Fructus Schizandrae Chinensis (*Wu Wei Zi*)

Additions & subtractions: If there is excessive phlegm and nausea, add Rhizoma Pinelliae Ternatae (*Ban Xia*). If there is abdominal distention, add Pericarpium Citri Reticulatae (*Chen Pi*) and Fructus Aurantii (*Zhi Ke*). If the patient is constitutionally weak, add Cordyceps Chinensis (*Dong Chong Xia Cao*). For severe coughing with facial edema, add Semen Pruni Armeniacae (*Xing Ren*). And for enduring cough that will not stop, add Radix Asteris Tatarici (*Zi Wan*) and Flos Tussilaginis Farfarae (*Kuan Dong Hua*).

Acupuncture & moxibustion: *Fei Shu* (Bl 13), *Pi Shu* (Bl 20), *Wei Shu* (Bl 21), *Zu San Li* (St 36), *Feng Long* (St 40), *San Yin Jiao* (Sp 6)

Key advice: Use moxa on *Pi Shu* and *Wei Shu* in order to supplement and warm spleen yang as opposed to only supplementing spleen qi since this is most definitely a cold phlegm condition due to yang vacuity.

See the phlegm rheum pattern below in the chapter on fluids and humors pattern discrimination for other treatment options.

Lung Qi Vacuity with Simultaneous Heat

Disease causes, disease mechanisms: Due to enduring heat in the lungs, qi is damaged and consumed. Therefore the lungs' lose their control over diffusion and downbearing, while heat stews the juices and engenders phlegm. Heat may also damage the network vessels resulting in hematemsis.

Main symptoms: Enduring coughing and wheezing, thick, yellow phlegm, coughing of pus and blood, vexatious heat in the chest, facial edema, and gradual weight loss

Tongue & coating: A thin, white or thin, yellow, slimy tongue coating

Pulse image: A floating, vacuous pulse especially at the inch position

Treatment principles: Supplement the qi and clear heat, transform phlegm and stop coughing

Rx: *Ren Shen Ge Jie San* (Ginseng & Gecko Powder)

Ingredients:

Gecko (*Ge Jie*)
Radix Panacis Ginseng (*Ren Shen*)
Sclerotium Poriae Cocos (*Fu Ling*)
Cortex Radicis Mori Albi (*Sang Bai Pi*)
Semen Pruni Armeniacae (*Xing Ren*)
Bulbus Fritillariae Cirrhosae (*Chuan Bei Mu*)
Rhizoma Anemarrhenae (*Zhi Mu*)
mix-fried Radix Glycyrrhizae (*Zhi Gan Cao*)

Acupuncture & moxibustion: *Fei Shu* (Bl 13), *Shan Zhong* (CV 17), *Chi Ze* (Lu 5), *Zu San Li* (St 36), *Feng Long* (St 40), *Guan Yuan* (CV 4)

Key advice: This is a commonly encountered pattern. There is simultaneous qi vacuity, heat, and phlegm.

Lung Dryness with Simultaneous Phlegm

Disease causes, disease mechanisms: This pattern is due to either enduring disease consuming lung fluids while still engendering phlegm or invasion by dryness and heat damaging fluids and engendering phlegm. However, dryness is not severe and yin is not yet vacuous.

Main symptoms: Dry cough with some thick, difficult to expectorate phlegm, wheezing, a dry, sore throat

Tongue & coating: A red, dry tongue with scanty coating

Pulse image: A rapid, fine but forceful pulse

Treatment principles: Moisten the lungs and clear heat, rectify the qi and transform phlegm

Rx: *Bei Mu Gua Lou San* (Fritillaria & Trichosanthes Powder)

Ingredients:

Bulbus Fritillariae (*Bei Mu*)
Fructus Trichosanthis Kirlowii (*Gua Lou*)
Radix Trichosanthis Kirlowii (*Tian Hua Fen*)
Sclerotium Poriae Cocos (*Fu Ling*)
Pericarpium Citri Erythrocarpae (*Ju Hong*)
Radix Platycodi Grandiflori (*Jie Geng*)

Additions & subtractions: For severe coughing and wheezing, add Semen Pruni Armeniacae (*Xing Ren*), Folium Eriobotryae Japonicae (*Pi Pa Ye*), and Flos Tussilaginis Farfarae (*Kuan Dong Hua*). For a simultaneous exterior condition, add Folium Mori Albi (*Sang Ye*), Semen Pruni Armeniacae (*Xing Ren*), Radix Peucedani (*Qian Hu*), and Fructus Arctii Lappae (*Niu Bang Zi*). For severe dryness and sore throat, add Radix Scrophulariae Ningpoensis (*Xuan Shen*), Tuber Ophiopogonis Japonicae (*Mai Dong*), and Rhizoma Anemarrhenae (*Zhi Mu*).

Acupuncture & moxibustion: *Fei Shu* (Bl 13), *Zhong Fu* (Lu 1), *Shan Zhong* (CV 17), *Feng Long* (St 40), *Chi Ze* (Lu 5)

Key advice: Phlegm and dryness may seem antithetical, but they are not. In clinical practice, dryness is always associated with some heat. Heat damages yin fluids but also stews the juices and engenders phlegm.

Lung Dryness, Large Intestine Blockage

Disease causes, disease mechanisms: If the lungs are damaged by dryness and heat, this may cause the lungs to lose their control over clearing and depurating. On the one hand, this may result in chest distention and cough with excessive phlegm. On the other, this may affect the lungs' diffusion of fluids. In this case, the large intestine may lose its nourishment, resulting in abdominal distention and constipation.

Main symptoms: Cough with excessive phlegm, chest and abdominal fullness and distention, constipation

Tongue & coating: A red tongue with scanty, dry, yellowish coating

Pulse image: A fine, wiry, rapid pulse, possibly floating in the inch positions

Treatment principles: Moisten dryness and transform phlegm, nourish the intestines and free the stools

Rx: *Wu Ren Ju Pi Tang* (Five [Ingredients] Seeds & Orange Peel Decoction)

Ingredients:

Semen Pruni Armeniacae (*Xing Ren*)
Semen Pruni (*Yu Li Ren*)
Semen Pruni Persicae (*Tao Ren*)
Semen Biotae Orientalis (*Bai Zi Ren*)
Pericarpium Citri Reticulatae (*Chen Pi*)

Acupuncture & moxibustion: *Da Zhui* (GV 14), *Shi Xuan* (M-UE-1-5), *He Gu* (LI 4), *Li Dui* (St 45), *Zu San Li* (St 36), *Feng Long* (St 40), *Tian Shu* (St 25)

Key advice: In four aspect or defensive, qi, constructive, blood pattern discrimination, this is categorized as a qi aspect pattern.

Lung Yin Debility & Consumption

Disease causes, disease mechanisms: Enduring heat in the lungs may eventually consume yin. This heat may be due to externally invading wind, heat, and dryness or to phlegm heat and heat toxins that have exhausted yin.

Main symptoms: Dry, unproductive cough, or cough with sticky phlegm, scanty in amount, possibly tinged with blood, chronic, low-grade sore throat, low-grade fever, dry nose, parched lips, raspy breathing resembling wheezing

Tongue & coating: A red tongue with a dry, scanty coating

Pulse image: A fine, rapid, commonly floating pulse in the inch position

Treatment principles: Enrich yin and moisten the lungs, stop coughing and transform phlegm

Rx: *Sha Shen Mai Men Dong Tang* (Glehnia & Ophiopogon Decoction)

Ingredients:

Radix Glehniae Littoralis (*Sha Shen*)
Tuber Ophiopogonis Japonicae (*Mai Dong*)
Rhizoma Polygonati Odorati (*Yu Zhu*)
Folium Mori Albi (*Sang Ye*)
Radix Trichosanthis Kirlowii (*Tian Hua Fen*)
Semen Dolichoris Lablabis (*Bai Bian Dou*)
Radix Glycyrrhizae (*Gan Cao*)

Additions & subtractions: If there is coughing and rapid breathing, add Fructus Schizandrae Chinensis (*Wu Wei Zi*) and Fructus Terminaliae Chebulae (*He Zi*). If there is tidal fever, add Radix Stellariae Dichotomae (*Yin Chai Hu*), Herba Artemisae Apiaceae (*Qing Hao*), Carapax Amydae Sinensis (*Bie Jia*), and Rhizoma Picrorrhizae (*Hu Huang Lian*). If there are night sweats, add Fructus Pruni Mume (*Wu Mei*) and Fructus Levis Tritici Aestivi (*Fu Xiao Mai*). If there is expectoration of yellow phlegm, add Concha Cyclinae Meretricis (*Hai Ge Ke*), Rhizoma Anemarrhenae (*Zhi Mu*), and Radix Scutellariae Baicalensis (*Huang Qin*). And if there is blood in the phlegm, add Cortex Radicis Moutan (*Dan Pi*), Fructus Gardeniae Jasminoidis (*Shan Zhi*), and Nodus Rhizomatis Nelumbinis Nuciferae (*Ou Jie*).

Acupuncture & moxibustion: *Lie Que* (Lu 7), *Zhao Hai* (Ki 6), *Zhong Fu* (Lu 1), *Fei Shu* (Bl 13)

Auxiliary points: If there is malar flushing and heat in the centers of the hands and feet, add *Tai Xi* (Ki 3) and *San Yin Jiao* (Sp 6).

Key advice: Because the authors live in a high altitude, arid climate, we commonly see this pattern. Chinese medicine treats it very effectively.

Lung Qi & Yin Vacuity

Disease causes, disease mechanisms: Again due to enduring disease, qi and yin have both been damaged. Thus there is dryness and loss of control over the diffusing and downbearing functions of the lungs.

Main symptoms: Headache, fever, hacking cough, wheezing, a dry nose and parched throat, chest oppression, lateral costal pain, easy anger and vexation, oral thirst

Tongue & coating: A dry tongue with scanty or no coating

Pulse image: A vacuous, large, rapid pulse

Treatment principles: Clear heat and moisten dryness, supplement the qi and nourish yin

Rx: *Qing Zao Jiu Fei Tang* (Clear Dryness & Rescue the Lungs Decoction)

Ingredients:

Folium Mori Albi (*Sang Ye*)
Gypsum Fibrosum (*Shi Gao*)
Tuber Ophiopogonis Japonicae (*Mai Dong*)
Gelatinum Corii Asini (*E Jiao*)
Semen Sesami Indici (*Hei Zhi Ma*)
Semen Pruni Armeniacae (*Xing Ren*)
mix-fried Folium Eriobotryae Japonicae (*Pi Pa Ye*)
Radix Panacis Ginseng (*Ren Shen*)
Radix Glycyrrhizae (*Gan Cao*)

Additions & subtractions: If there is excessive, thick, sticky phlegm, add Bulbus Fritillariae Cirrhosae (*Chuan Bei Mu*) and Semen Trichosanthis Kirlowii (*Gua Lou Ren*). If there is blood-streaked phlegm, add uncooked Radix Rehmanniae (*Sheng Di*) and Cacumen Biotae Orientalis (*Ce Bai Ye*). And if there is simultaneous constipation with dry, bound stools, add Semen Pruni Persicae (*Tao Ren*) and Semen Cannabis Sativae (*Hua Ma Ren*).

Acupuncture & moxibustion: *Fei Shu* (Bl 13), *Zhong Fu* (Lu 1), *Shan Zhong* (CV 17), *Lie Que* (Lu 7), *Zhao Hai* (Ki 6), *Zu San Li* (St 36)

Key advice: Because of the interrelationship of the yin and qi, dual qi and yin vacuity is commonly seen in clinical practice. The above formula also presupposes the presence of evil heat continuing to damage qi and yin and thus the pulse is large.

Lung Qi & Yin Vacuity with Phlegm & Heat

Disease causes, disease mechanisms: Due to enduring disease, heat has damaged and consumed lung qi and yin while at the same time engendering phlegm.

Main symptoms: Enduring lung disease, low-grade fever, thick, yellow, difficult to expectorate phlegm, dry, itchy, sore throat, hoarseness, persistent cough, dry mouth, oral thirst

Tongue & coating: A red tongue with dry, scanty, yellow coating

Pulse image: A rapid, surging, slippery pulse

Treatment principles: Moisten the lungs and supplement the qi, clear heat and transform phlegm

Rx: *Qing Fei Tang* (Clear the Lungs Decoction)

Ingredients:

Tuber Ophiopogonis Japonicae (*Mai Dong*)
Tuber Asparagi Cochinensis (*Tian Dong*)
Fructus Schizandrae Chinensis (*Wu Wei Zi*)
Sclerotium Poriae Cocos (*Fu Ling*)
Radix Angelicae Sinensis (*Dang Gui*)
Radix Scutellariae Baicalensis (*Huang Qin*)
Fructus Gardeniae Jasminoidis (*Shan Zhi*)
Caulis Bambusae In Taeniis (*Zhu Ru*)
Cortex Radicis Mori Albi (*Sang Bai Pi*)
Semen Armeniacae (*Xing Ren*)
Bulbus Fritillariae (*Bei Mu*)
Radix Platycodi Grandiflori (*Jie Geng*)
Pericarpium Citri Reticulatae (*Chen Pi*)
Fructus Zizyphi Jujubae (*Da Zao*)
uncooked Rhizoma Zingiberis (*Sheng Jiang*)
Radix Glycyrrhizae (*Gan Cao*)

Acupuncture & moxibustion: *Fei Shu* (Bl 13), *Zhong Fu* (Lu 1), *Shan Zhong* (CV 17), *Chi Ze* (Lu 5), *Feng Long* (St. 40), *Zu San Li* (St 36), *San Yin Jiao* (Sp 6)

Key advice: This is also a very commonly seen pattern in clinical practice. It is complex in the way that real-life patients typically are.

Lung/Kidney Yin Vacuity

Disease causes, disease mechanisms: Due to insufficient natural endowment, aging, or enduring disease, either kidney yin vacuity may give rise to simultaneous lung yin vacuity or vice versa.

Main symptoms: Dry cough with scanty phlegm, chronic, low-grade sore throat, afternoon malar flushing, possible night sweats and tidal fever, low back and knee soreness and weakness, polyuria, nocturia

Tongue & coating: A red tongue with scanty coating

Pulse image: Fine and floating

Treatment principles: Supplement the kidneys and moisten the lungs, transform phlegm and stop coughing

Rx: *Bai He Gu Jin Tang* (Lily Secure Metal Decoction)

Ingredients:

Bulbus Lilii (*Bai He*)
uncooked Radix Rehmanniae (*Sheng Di*)
prepared Radix Rehmanniae (*Shu Di*)
Tuber Ophiopogonis Japonici (*Mai Men Dong*)
Radix Scrophulariae Ningpoensis (*Xuan Shen*)
Bulbus Fritillariae (*Bei Mu*)
Radix Platycodi Grandiflori (*Jie Geng*)
Radix Angelicae Sinensis (*Dang Gui*)
Radix Albus Paeoniae Lactiflorae (*Bai Shao*)
Radix Glycyrrhizae (*Gan Cao*)

Additions & subtractions: For excessive phlegm, add Semen Trichosanthis Kirlowii (*Gua Lou Ren*) and Cortex Radicis Mori Albi (*Sang Bai Pi*). For coughing blood, remove Platycodon and add Rhizoma Imperatae Cyclindricae (*Bai Mao Gen*) and Herba

Agrimoniae Pilosae (*He Xian Cao*). For high fever and dark yellow phlegm, add Rhizoma Anemarrhenae (*Zhi Mu*) and Herba Cum Radice Houttuyniae Cordatae (*Yu Xing Cao*).

Acupuncture & moxibustion: *Fei Shu* (Bl 13), *Shen Shu* (Bl 23), *San Yin Jiao* (Sp 6), *Zhao Hai* (Ki 6), *Lie Que* (Lu 7)

Lung/Kidney Yang Vacuity

Disease causes, disease mechanisms: Due to insufficient natural endowment, enduring disease, and aging, there is lung qi vacuity and kidney yang vacuity.

Main symptoms: Cough with clear, watery phlegm, cough aggravated by exertion or talking, difficult breathing, inability to lie flat, chest oppression, heart fluster, cold body, sweating, a somber white facial complexion, fear of chill, fatigued spirit, exhaustion, no thirst

Tongue & coating: A pale or dark, purplish tongue with a thin, glossy coating

Pulse image: A deep, fine, forceless, faint or bound, regularly intermittent pulse

Treatment principles: Supplement the lungs and grasp the kidneys, downbear the qi and stabilize dyspnea

Rx: *Ding Chuan Gu Ben Tang* (Stabilize Dyspnea & Secure the Root Decoction) plus *Bu Fei Tang* (Supplement the Lungs Decoction) with additions & subtractions

Ingredients:

Radix Astragali Membranacei (*Huang Qi*)
Radix Panacis Ginseng (*Ren Shen*)
mix-fried Radix Glycyrrhizae (*Zhi Gan Cao*)
Cordyceps Chinensis (*Dong Chong Xia Cao*)
prepared Radix Rehmanniae (*Shu Di*)
Semen Juglandis Regiae (*Hu Tao Rou*)
Fructus Schizandrae Chinensis (*Wu Wei Zi*)
Magnetitum (*Ling Ci Shi*)
Lignum Aquilariae Agallochae (*Chen Xiang*)
Radix Asteris Tatarici (*Zi Wan*)

Flos Tussilaginis Farfarae (*Kuan Dong*)
Fructus Perillae Frutescentis (*Su Zi*)
lime-processed Rhizoma Pinelliae Ternatae (*Fa Ban Xia*)
Pericarpium Citri Erythrocarpae (*Ju Hong*)

Additions & subtractions: If there is lung vacuity with cold, fear of chill, and a pale tongue, add Cortex Cinnamomi (*Rou Gui*), dry Rhizoma Zingiberis (*Gan Jiang*), and Stalactitum (*Zhong Ru Shi*). If yin is simultaneously damaged with low-grade fever, and there is a red tongue with scanty coating, add Tuber Ophiopogonis Japonicae (*Mai Dong*), Rhizoma Polygonati Odorati (*Yu Zhu*), and uncooked Radix Rehmanniae (*Sheng Di*). If there is qi vacuity with stasis obstruction, add Radix Angelicae Sinensis (*Dang Gui*), Radix Salviae Miltiorrhizae (*Dan Shen*), and Lignum Sappan (*Su Mu*).

Acupuncture & moxibustion: *Fei Shu* (Bl 13), *Tai Yuan* (Lu 9), *Guan Yuan* (CV 4), *Shen Shu* (Bl 23), *Ming Men* (GV 4), *Gao Huang Shu* (Bl 43)

Key advice: Have the patient burn numerous tiny cones of moxa on *Guan Yuan* daily.

Lung Network Vessel Stasis & Obstruction

Disease causes, disease mechanisms: In cases of enduring coughing of phlegm and expectorating of blood, the network vessels may be damaged and blood may spill over. This then obstructs and hinders the lung network vessels. This may also be due to enduring deep-lying phlegm congesting in and obstructing the lungs. Thus the qi of the lungs becomes congested and the blood becomes static.

Main symptoms: Cough with expectoration of phlegm, dark, purplish blood clots within the phlegm, possible coughing and then vomiting up blood clots, heart palpitations, chest oppression, piercing pain, cough making lying down difficult, bluish purple lips, a dark, dusky face, dark rings around the eyes

Tongue & coating: A purple, dark tongue or static patches

Pulse image: Deep, wiry, and choppy; wiry and slow; or bound and regularly intermittent

Treatment principles: Quicken the blood and transform stasis, free the network vessels and stop bleeding

Rx: *Xue Fu Zhu Yu Tang* (Blood Mansion Dispel Stasis Decoction)

Ingredients:

Semen Pruni Persicae (*Tao Ren*)
Flos Carthami Tinctorii (*Hong Hua*)
Radix Angelicae Sinensis (*Dang Gui*)
Radix Ligustici Wallichii (*Chuan Xiong*)
Radix Rubrus Paeoniae Lactiflorae (*Chi Shao*)
Radix Acyranthis Bidentatae (*Niu Xi*)
Radix Bupleuri (*Chai Hu*)
Radix Platycodi Grandiflori (*Jie Geng*)
Fructus Aurantii (*Zhi Ke*)
uncooked Radix Rehmanniae (*Sheng Di*)
Radix Glycyrrhizae (*Gan Cao*)

Acupuncture & moxibustion: *Fei Shu* (Bl 13), *Ge Shu* (Bl 17), *Shan Zhong* (CV 17), *Qi Men* (Liv 14), *Xue Hai* (Sp 10)

Key advice: Blood stasis may complicate cold rheum and vacuity cold conditions. In that case, one should add some appropriate blood-quickening and stasis-transforming medicinals to the guiding formula as in the lung/kidney yang vacuity modifications above.

Patients with this pattern usually are seriously ill. Therefore, they should be referred to a Western physician for diagnosis. They may have cardiopulmonary disease or lung cancer.

Intestinal Vacuity Not Securing

Disease causes, disease mechanisms: This pattern is due to enduring disease in turn due to spleen vacuity which eventually reaches the kidneys and affects the astringing, closing function of the kidney qi.

Main symptoms: Enduring diarrhea and dysentery, prolapsed rectum, fecal incontinence, mild, persistent abdominal pain that diminishes in response to pressure and warmth, fatigued spirit, lack of strength, a sallow yellow or somber white facial complexion, scanty appetite, low back and leg soreness and weakness

Tongue & coating: A pale tongue with a thin, white coating

Pulse image: A fine, slow pulse

Treatment principles: Warm the center and supplement vacuity, secure the intestines and stop diarrhea

Rx: *Zhen Ren Yang Zang Tang* (True Person Nourish the Viscera Decoction)

Ingredients:

Radix Panacis Ginseng (*Ren Shen*)
Radix Angelicae Sinensis (*Dang Gui*)
Rhizoma Atractylodis Macrocephalae (*Bai Zhu*)
Semen Myristicae Fragrantis (*Rou Dou Kou*)
Cortex Cinnamomi (*Rou Gui*)
Radix Glycyrrhizae (*Gan Cao*)
Radix Albus Paeoniae Lactiflorae (*Bai Shao*)
Radix Auklandiae (*Mu Xiang*)
Fructus Terminaliae Chebulae (*He Zi*)
Pericarpium Papaveris Sominiferae (*Ying Su Ke*)

Additions & subtractions: For rectal prolapse, add Radix Astragali Membranacei (*Huang Qi*) and Rhizoma Cimicifugae (*Sheng Ma*). For diarrhea with undigested food in the stools and chilled extremities, add Radix Praeparatus Aconiti Carmichaeli (*Fu Zi*) and dry Rhizoma Zingiberis (*Gan Jiang*). For tenesmus, add Semen Arecae Catechu (*Bing Lang*).

Acupuncture & moxibustion: *Zu San Li* (St 36), *San Yin Jiao* (Sp 6), *Zhong Wan* (CV 12), *Tian Shu* (St 25), *Qi Hai* (CV 6), *Pi Shu* (Bl 20), *Wei Shu* (Bl 21), *Shen Shu* (Bl 23), *Hui Yang* (Bl 35)

Auxiliary points: If there is rectal prolapse, add *Bai Hui* (GV 20).

Key advice: This pattern is an evolution of spleen/kidney yang vacuity diarrhea or dysentery. In this case, the kidney qi is no longer astringing and securing as it should. Whenever diarrhea has gone on for a long period of time, one should consider adding some astringent medicinals, even if some other mechanism is at work as well.

Excessive Fire in the Large Intestine

Disease causes, disease mechanisms: This pattern is due to overeating acrid, hot, peppery foods, greasy, fatty, fried foods, and drinking too much alcohol or invasion of the *yang ming* by evil heat.

Main symptoms: Constipation, brownish, watery stool, a burning sensation around the anus, high fever, epigastric glomus and fullness, pain in the abdomen that dislikes pressure, if severe, tidal fever, delirious speech, and profuse sweating from the hands and feet

Tongue & coating: A yellow, prickly tongue coating that may even be charred black and dry

Pulse image: A deep, replete pulse

Treatment principles: Greatly drain heat accumulation from the large intestine

Rx: *Da Cheng Qi Tang* (Great Order the Qi Decoction)

Ingredients:

Radix Et Rhizoma Rhei (*Da Huang*)
Cortex Magnoliae Officinalis (*Hou Po*)
Fructus Immaturus Aurantii (*Zhi Shi*)
Mirabilitum (*Mang Xiao*)

Additions & subtractions: If *yang ming* bowel repletion is relatively mild or there is mild damage of fluids and humors, subtract Mirabilitum. This results in *Xiao Cheng Qi Tang* (Minor Order the Qi Decoction). If there is severe fluid dryness of the intestines as manifested by constipation, subtract Magnolia and Citrus Immaturus and add Radix Scrophulariae Ningpoensis (*Yuan Shen*), uncooked Radix Rehmanniae (*Sheng Di*), and Tuber Ophiopogonis Japanicae (*Mai Men Dong*). This results in *Zeng Ye Cheng Qi Tang* (Increase Fluids & Order the Qi Decoction). If there is no glomus or abdominal fullness but mild constipation with irritability and a slippery, rapid pulse, subtract Citrus Immaturus and Magnolia and add mix-fried Radix Glycyrrhizae (*Zhi Gan Cao*). This results in *Tiao Wei Cheng Qi Tang* (Regulate the Stomach Order the Qi Decoction).

Acupuncture & moxibustion: *Tian Shu* (St 25), *Zu San Li* (St 36), *Da Chang Shu* (Bl 25), *Da Zhui* (GV 14), *Qu Chi* (LI 11), *He Gu* (LI 4), *Zhi Gou* (TB 6)

Large Intestine Vacuity Cold

Disease cause, disease mechanisms: Due to enduring disease, aging, or constitutional weakness, spleen and stomach yang is vacuous and weak and thus also the large intestine. Therefore the transportation and transformation of fluids is affected.

Main symptoms: Pain in the abdomen, borborygmus, loose stool, clear, copious urine

Tongue & coating: A pale, swollen tongue with a thin, white, moist coating

Pulse image: A deep, slow pulse

Treatment principles: Fortify the spleen and seep dampness, scatter cold and stop diarrhea

Rx: *Wei Ling San* (Stomach Poria Powder)

Ingredients:

Rhizoma Atractylodis (*Cang Zhu*)
Cortex Magnoliae Officinalis (*Hou Po*)
Pericarpium Citri Reticulatae (*Chen Pi*)
Sclerotium Poriae Cocos (*Fu Ling*)
Sclerotium Polypori Umbellati (*Zhu Ling*)
Rhizoma Atractylodis Macrocephalae (*Bai Zhu*)
Rhizoma Alismatis (*Ze Xie*)
Ramulus Cinnamomi (*Gui Zhi*)
Radix Glycyrrhizae (*Gan Cao*)
uncooked Rhizoma Zingiberis (*Sheng Jiang*)
Fructus Zizyphi Jujubae (*Da Zao*)

Acupuncture & moxibustion: *Tian Shu* (St 25), *Zu San Li* (St 36), *Shang Ju Xu* (St 37), *Zhong Wan* (CV 12), *Shui Fen* (CV 9), *Pi Shu* (Bl 20), *Da Chang Shu* (Bl 25)

Key advice: This pattern is essentially the same as spleen yang vacuity except that there is more pronounced disturbance of water metabolism even to the point of urinary difficulty.

Large Intestine Damp Heat

Disease causes, disease mechanisms: Due to overeating sweet, fatty, thick-flavored foods, dampness may accumulate in the body. If evil dampness becomes depressed and endures for a long time, it may transform into heat. However, it may transform into heat even quicker and more surely if the patient eats acrid, hot, peppery foods or drinks alcohol.

Main symptoms: Constipation or damp heat diarrhea (as in chronic colitis), reddish urine, burning heat around the anus, torpid intake, abdominal distention, sores in the mouth, acne with swollen, red lesions in the *yang ming* area of the face

Tongue & coating: A yellow, slimy tongue coating

Pulse image: A slippery, rapid pulse

Treatment principles: Clear heat, transform dampness, open the bowels

Rx: *Bai Tou Weng Tang* (Pulsatilla Decoction)

Ingredients:

Radix Pulsatillae Chinensis (*Bai Tou Weng*)
Rhizoma Coptidis Chinensis (*Huang Lian*)
Cortex Phellodendri (*Huang Bai*)
Cortex Fraxini (*Qin Pi*)

Additions & subtractions: If there is damp heat diarrhea or dysentery and heat is severe, add Cortex Radicis Moutan (*Dan Pi*), Radix Rubrus Paeoniae Lactiflorae (*Chi Shao*), Caulis Sargentodoxae (*Hong Teng*), and/or Herba Patriniae Heterophyllae (*Bai Jiang Cao*). If dampness is more severe, add Rhizoma Atractylodis (*Cang Zhu*), Semen Coicis Lachryma-jobi (*Yi Ren*), and Semen Plantaginis (*Che Qian Zi*). If there is constipation, add *Yin Chen Hao Tang* (Artemisia Capillaris Decoction): Herba Artemisiae Capillaris (*Yin Chen Hao*), Fructus Gardeniae Jasminoidis (*Zhi Zi*), Radix Et Rhizoma

111

Rhei (*Da Huang*). If there is concomitant yin vacuity due to damage by smoldering damp heat, add Tuber Ophiopogonis Japonicae (*Mai Dong*) and Radix Glehniae Littoralis (*Sha Shen*).

Acupuncture & moxibustion: *Nei Ting* (St 44), *Qu Chi* (LI 11), *Yin Ling Quan* (Sp 9), *Zhong Wan* (CV 12), *Tian Shu* (St 25), *Zhong Ji* (CV 3), *Da Chang Shu* (Bl 25)

Auxiliary points: For bloody stools, add *Xue Hai* (Sp 10). For mucus in the stools, add *Shang Qiu* (Sp 5), *Feng Long* (St 40), and *Pi Shu* (Bl 20).

Key advice: If there is a slippery, rapid pulse and there is diarrhea or dysentery, use this formula even if the patient appears constitutionally vacuous. It is also important that patients avoid foods that contain a lot of sugar or sweets, acrid, hot, peppery foods, alcohol, or foods made through fermentations, including bread and vinegar.

Large Intestine Conduction & Conveyance Loses Its Duty, Dampness & Turbidity Cloud Above

Disease causes, disease mechanisms: If evil dampness disturbs the functions of conveyance and conduction of the large intestine below, upbearing of the clear and downbearing of the turbid are not separated. Thus turbid dampness accumulates and is upborne.

Main symptoms: Headache and distention, bodily heaviness, nausea and vomiting, difficult urination, thirst but drinking causes more nausea and vomiting

Tongue & coating: A slimy, white tongue coating

Pulse image: Soggy, wiry pulse

Treatment principles: First, open the portals by means of penetrating aromatics, secondly eliminate dampness

Rx: *Su He Xiang Wan* (Liquid Styrax Pills) plus *Fu Ling Pi Tang* (Cortex Poriae Decoction)

Ingredients:

Su He Xiang Wan:

Rhizoma Atractylodis Macrocephalae (*Bai Zhu*)
clear Radix Auklandiae (*Qing Mu Xiang*)
Cornu Rhinocerotis (*Wu Xi Jiao*)
Rhizoma Cyperi Rotundi (*Xiang Fu*)
Cinnabar (*Zhu Sha*)
Fructus Terminaliae Chebulae (*He Zi*)
Lignum Santali Albi (*Bai Tan Xiang*)
Lignum Aquilariae Agallochae (*Chen Xiang*)
Benzoinum (*An Xi Xiang*)
Secretio Moschi Moschiferi (*She Xiang*)
Flos Caryophylli (*Ding Xiang*)
Fructus Piperis Longi (*Bi Ba*)
Borneolum (*Long Nao*)
Oleum Stryracis Liquidis (*Su He Xiang You*)
Resina Olibani (*Ru Xiang*)

Fu Ling Pi Tang:

Cortex Sclerotii Poriae Cocos (*Fu Ling Pi*)
Semen Coicis Lachryma-jobi (*Yi Yi Ren*)
Sclerotium Polypori Umbellati (*Zhu Ling*)
Pericarpium Arecae Catechu (*Da Fu Pi*)
Medulla Tetrapanacis Papyriferi (*Deng Xin Cao*)
Herba Lophatheri Gracilis (*Dan Zhu Ye*)

Acupuncture & moxibustion: *Zu San Li* (St 36), *San Yin Jiao* (Sp 6), *Feng Long* (St 40), *Nei Ting* (St 44), *Bai Hui* (GV 20)

Key advice: Although this is titled a large intestine pattern, it is usually categorized under triple burner pattern discrimination as a middle burner pattern.

Dampness Obstructing the Intestinal Tract, Conduction & Conveyance Lose Their Command

Disease causes, disease mechanisms: Enduring damp heat may obstruct the flow of qi in the intestines, causing fullness and distention in the lower abdomen and difficulty defecating. If dampness is upborne, this may result in clouding of the spirit.

Main symptoms: Clouded spirit, lower abdominal fullness and distention, difficulty defecating

Tongue & coating: A slimy, turbid tongue coating

Pulse image: A slippery, rapid pulse

Treatment principles: Disinhibit the qi and dispel obstruction, eliminate dampness and abduct turbidity

Rx: *Xuan Qing Dao Zhuo Tang* (Return the Clear & Abduct the Turbid Decoction)

Ingredients:

Sclerotium Polypori Umbellati (*Zhu Ling*)
Sclerotium Poriae Cocos (*Fu Ling*)
Calcitum (*Han Shui Shi*)
Excrementum Bombycis Mori (*Can Sha*)
Fructus Gleditschiae Chinensis (*Zao Jiao*)

Acupuncture & moxibustion: *Tian Shu* (St 25), *Shang Ju Xu* (St 37), *Xia Ju Xu* (St 39), *Zu San Li* (St 36), *Nei Ting* (St 44), *San Yin Jiao* (Sp 6)

Key advice: This pattern is likewise categorized by triple burner pattern discrimination as a middle burner pattern.

Large Intestine Fluid Consumption

Disease causes, disease mechanisms: Due to aging, enduring disease, or the sequelae of a warm disease, blood and yin may be vacuous and scanty and, therefore, so may large intestine fluids.

Main symptoms: Constipation with dry, bound stools, a sallow yellow, lusterless facial complexion, oral thirst, headache, vertigo, heart palpitations, pale, dry lips

Tongue & coating: A pale, dry tongue

Pulse image: A fine pulse

Treatment principles: Nourish the blood and moisten dryness

Rx: *Run Chang Wan* (Moisten the Intestines Pills)

Ingredients:

Semen Cannabis Sativae (*Huo Ma Ren*)
Semen Pruni Persicae (*Tao Ren*)
Radix Angelicae Sinensis (*Dang Gui*)
uncooked Radix Rehmanniae (*Sheng Di*)
Fructus Aurantii (*Zhi Ke*)
Honey (*Bai Mi*)

Additions & subtractions: If there are signs of vacuity heat, add Rhizoma Anemarrhenae (*Zhi Mu*) and Rhizoma Polygonati Odorati (*Yu Zhu*). If yin vacuity signs are more severe with vexatious heat in the five hearts and a red tongue, add Radix Scrophulariae Ningpoensis (*Xuan Shen*), Tuber Ophiopogonis Japonicae (*Mai Dong*), and uncooked Radix Polygoni Multiflori (*Shou Wu*).

Acupuncture & moxibustion: *Ge Shu* (Bl 17), *Pi Shu* (Bl 20), *Shen Shu* (Bl 23), *Da Chang Shu* (Bl 25), *Tian Shu* (St 25), *San Yin Jiao* (Sp 6), *Zu San Li* (St 36), *Guan Yuan* (CV 4)

Key advice: If fluids have already recovered but the stools are still dry and bound, use *Wu Ren Wan* (Five Seeds Pills): Semen Pruni Persicae (*Tao Ren*), Semen Pruni

Armeniacae (*Xing Ren*), Semen Biotae Orientalis (*Bai Zi Ren*), Semen Pini (*Song Zi Ren*), Semen Pruni (*Yu Li Ren*), Pericarpium Citri Reticulatae (*Chen Pi*).

Large Intestine Qi Stagnation

Disease causes, disease mechanisms: If there is a weak spleen, overeating may lead to food stagnation, which thus depresses the qi of the intestines. This then results in abdominal distention and fullness.

Main symptoms: Epigastric and lower abdominal distention and fullness, pain that refuses pressure, constipation, nausea

Tongue & coating: A slimy tongue coating

Pulse image: A slippery pulse

Treatment principles: Supplement the spleen and disperse accumulations

Rx: *Zhi Zhu Wan* (Citrus & Atractylodes Pills)

Ingredients:

Rhizoma Atractylodis Macrocephalae (*Bai Zhu*)
Fructus Immaturus Aurantii (*Zhi Shi*)

Additions & subtractions: For nausea and lack of appetite, add Massa Medica Fermentata (*Shen Qu*) and Fructus Germinatus Hordei Vulgaris (*Mai Ya*). For oppression and fullness, add Pericarpium Citri Reticulatae (*Chen Pi*) and Rhizoma Pinelliae Ternatae (*Ban Xia*).

Acupuncture & moxibustion: *Zhong Wan* (CV 12), *Tian Shu* (St 25), *Zu San Li* (St 36), *He Gu* (LI 4), *Da Chang Shu* (Bl 25)

Key advice: This pattern is very similar to stomach food stagnation. However, the symptoms of abdominal distention and fullness are more pronounced. Based on the above formula, a certain amount of spleen vacuity is presupposed.

Large Intestine Heat Stasis

Disease causes, disease mechanisms: Overeating in general and overeating greasy, fatty foods and/or raw, chilled foods in particular can cause qi stagnation and blood stasis in the intestines. This qi stagnation may then give rise to transformative heat and the accumulation of dampness, which then combine to form damp heat. Thus there is dampness and heat mutually binding with stasis and stagnation.

Main symptoms: Severe, fixed pain in the lower abdomen that is worsened by pressure, localized heat, either constipation or mild diarrhea

Tongue & coating: Red with a yellow, slimy coating

Pulse image: Slippery and rapid or tight

Treatment principles: Clear heat and disinhibit dampness, quicken the blood and dispel stasis

Rx: *Yi Yi Fu Zi Bai Jiang San* (Coix, Aconite & Patrinia Powder)

Ingredients:

Semen Coicis Lachryma-jobi (*Yi Yi Ren*)
Radix Lateralis Praeparatus Aconiti Carmichaeli (*Fu Zi*)
Herba Patriniae Heterophyllae (*Bai Jiang Cao*)

Additions & subtractions: If there are no signs of cold, remove the Aconite. For more severe blood stasis, add Cortex Radicis Moutan (*Dan Pi*) and Semen Pruni Persicae (*Tao Ren*).

Acupuncture & moxibustion: *Lan Wei Xue* (M-LE-13), *He Gu* (LI 4), *Qu Chi* (LI 11), *Tian Shu* (St 25)

Key advice: This pattern describes acute appendicitis or intestinal abscess. Therefore, if there is any question about the patient's diagnosis or response to treatment, they should be referred to a Western physician.

Aconite is included in this formula because this pattern is often complicated by an element of cold. This goes along with Li Dong-yuan's observation that damp heat in the lower burner damages the liver and kidneys and leads to kidney yang vacuity and well as qi stagnation, blood stasis.

Kidney & Bladder Patterns

Kidney Qi Vacuity

Disease causes, disease mechanisms: The kidney qi may be vacuous and weak due to constitutional insufficiency, again, or enduring disease.

Main symptoms: Low back and knee soreness and weakness, loose teeth, loss of hair, impotence, seminal emission, uterine prolapse accompanied by weakness of the low back, frequent urination, nocturia, tinnitus, dizziness, diminished auditory acuity

Tongue & coating: A pale red tongue

Pulse image: A deep, weak pulse

Treatment principles: Supplement the kidneys and boost the qi

Rx: *Da Bu Yuan Jian* (Greatly Supplement the Origin Decoction)

Ingredients:

Radix Panacis Ginseng (*Ren Shen*)
Radix Dioscoreae Oppositae (*Shan Yao*)
prepared Radix Rehmanniae (*Shu Di*)
Cortex Eucommiae Ulmoidis (*Du Zhong*)
Radix Angelicae Sinensis (*Dang Gui*)
Fructus Corni Officinalis (*Shan Zhu Yu*)
Fructus Lycii Chinensis (*Gou Qi Zi*)
mix-fried Radix Glycyrrhizae (*Zhi Gan Cao*)

Acupuncture & moxibustion: *Shen Shu* (Bl 23), *Guan Yuan* (CV 4), *Zhi Shi* (Bl 52), *Zu San Li* (St 36), *Qi Hai* (CV 6)

Key advice: This pattern is not commonly seen in clinical practice. Most often, one sees kidney yin vacuity, kidney yang vacuity, or kidney qi not securing.

Kidneys Not Securing the Essence

Disease causes, disease mechanisms: This pattern is most often due to aging and enduring disease, which damage the kidney qi's function of closing and storing.

Main symptoms: Nocturia, enuresis, frequent, clear urination, spermatorrhea, premature ejaculation, low back and knee soreness and weakness

Tongue & coating: A pale tongue

Pulse image: A deep, fine pulse

Treatment principles: In case of frequent emission, supplement the kidneys and secure the essence. In case of enuresis, warm the kidneys and secure the qi

Rx: *Ji Sheng Mi Jing Wan* (*Aid to the Living* Secrete the Essence Pills)

Ingredients:

Semen Cuscutae (*Tu Si Zi*)
Concha Ostreae (*Mu Li*)
Os Draconis (*Long Gu*)
Fructus Schisandrae Chinensis (*Wu Wei Zi*)
Ootheca Mantidis (*Sang Piao Xiao*)
Radix Panacis Ginseng (*Ren Shen*)
Hallyositum Rubrum (*Chi Shi Zhi*)
Sclerotium Poriae Cocos (*Fu Ling*)

Additions & subtractions: For nocturnal emission and spermatorrhea, add Fructus Rosae Laevigatae (*Jin Ying Zi*), Stamen Nelumbinis Nuciferae (*Lian Xu*), Radix Polygalae Tenuifoliae (*Yuan Zhi*), Cortex Phellodendri (*Huang Bai*), Fructus Amomi (*Sha Ren*), and Radix Glycyrrhizae (*Gan Cao*). For frequent, long, clear urination and emaciation, add Fructus Psoraleae Corylifoliae (*Bu Gu Zi*) and Cornu Parvum Cervi (*Lu Rong*).

Acupuncture & moxibustion: *Shen Shu* (Bl 23), *Zhong Ji* (CV 3), *Guan Yuan* (CV 4), *San Yin Jiao* (Sp 6), *Zhi Shi* (Bl 52), *Zu San Li* (St 36)

Auxiliary points: For abnormal vaginal discharge that is clear like egg whites, add *Yin Ling Quan* (Sp 9).

Key advice: Do not use the astringing, securing method if polyuria, spermatorrhea, or abnormal vaginal discharge are due to heat.

Kidneys Not Astringing the Intestines

Disease causes, disease mechanisms: If diarrhea or dysentery endure for a long time, the kidney qi may fail to secure the intestines and perform their function of closing and storing. In that case, there will be unstopping diarrhea.

Main symptoms: Fifth watch diarrhea (*i.e.*, cock-crow diarrhea), no thought for food or drink, prolonged diarrhea that will not heal, abdominal pain, low back soreness, chilled extremities, fatigued spirit, lack of strength

Tongue & coating: A pale tongue

Pulse image: A deep, slow, forceless pulse

Treatment principles: Warm and supplement the kidneys, astringe the intestines and stop diarrhea

Rx: *Si Shen Wan* (Four Spirits Pills)

Ingredients:

Semen Myristicae Fragrantis (*Rou Dou Kou*)
Fructus Psoraleae Corylifoliae (*Bu Gu Zhi*)
Fructus Schizandrae Chinensis (*Wu Wei Zi*)
Fructus Evodiae Rutecarpae (*Wu Zhu Yu*)
uncooked Rhizoma Zingiberis (*Sheng Jiang*)
Fructus Zizyphi Jujubae (*Da Zao*)

Additions & subtractions: For cold hands and feet, add Radix Lateralis Praeparatus Aconiti Carmichaeli (*Fu Zi*) and Cortex Cinnamomi (*Rou Gui*). For rectal prolapse, add Radix Astragali Membranacei (*Huang Qi*) and Rhizoma Cimicifugae (*Sheng Ma*). For lower abdominal pain, subtract Evodia and Schizandra and add Radix Auklandiae (*Mu Xiang*) and Fructus Foeniculi Vulgaris (*Xiao Hui Xiang*).

Acupuncture & moxibustion: *Shen Shu* (Bl 23), *Guan Yuan* (CV 4), *Tian Shu* (St 25), *Zu San Li* (St 36), *Ming Men* (GV 4)

Key advice: Kidney qi not astringing the intestines may complicate other patterns of enduring diarrhea or dysentery. In that case, astringent medicinals are added to other guiding formulas based on other main patterns. The addition of astringents, such as Myristica can spell the difference between successful and unsuccessful treatment of chronic diarrhea. However, astringents should not be used to treat damp heat diarrhea or dysentery.

Kidneys Not Absorbing the Qi

Disease causes, disease mechanisms: If coughing and panting or wheezing endure for a long time or if the patient is constitutionally vacuous and weak, the kidney qi may fail to grasp or absorb the qi downborne by the lungs. Thus the qi counterflows back upward.

Main symptoms: Enduring cough, shortness of breath, panting and wheezing, trouble inhaling but no trouble exhaling, inability to breathe freely when lying down flat

Tongue & coating: A pale tongue with a thin, white coating

Pulse image: A deep, fine pulse

Treatment principles: In case of panting, supplement the kidneys to absorb the qi. In case of wheezing, supplement the kidneys and absorb the qi to stop asthma.

Rx: *Jin Gui Shen Qi Wan* (*Golden Cabinet* Kidney Qi Pills)

Ingredients:

prepared Radix Rehmanniae (*Shu Di*)
Fructus Corni Officinalis (*Shan Zhu Yu*)
Radix Dioscoreae Oppositae (*Shan Yao*)
Rhizoma Alismatis (*Ze Xie*)
Sclerotium Poriae Cocos (*Fu Ling*)
Cortex Radicis Moutan (*Dan Pi*)
Ramulus Cinnamomi (*Gui Zi*)
Radix Lateralis Praeparatus Aconiti Carmichaeli (*Fu Zi*)

Additions & subtractions: If there is cough with phlegm and severe asthma, add Hallyositum Rubrum (*Chi Shi*), Radix Panacis Ginseng (*Ren Shen*), and Fructus Schizandrae Chinensis (*Wu Wei Zi*). For asthma with palpitations and dizziness, add Hallyositum Rubrum and Schizandra and increase the dosage of Poria.

Acupuncture & moxibustion: *Shen Shu* (Bl 23), *Fei Shu* (Bl 13), *Ding Chuan* (M-BW-1b), *Gao Huang Shu* (Bl 43), *Zu San Li* (St 36), *Tai Xi* (Ki 3), *Tai Yuan* (Lu 9), *Qi Hai* (CV 6)

Key advice: Similar to the above pattern, kidneys not grasping the qi may complicate other patterns of enduring coughing and wheezing. In that case, astringents are added to the guiding formulas for those other patterns.

Kidney Yang Vacuity & Debility

Disease causes, disease mechanisms: This pattern is usually due to insufficient natural endowment, aging, or enduring disease. However, it may also be due to excessive sex and use of drugs.

Main symptoms: Low back and knee soreness and weakness, a cold feeling in the lower half of the body, lower abdominal tension, inhibited or excessive urination, nocturia, cock-crow diarrhea

Tongue & coating: A pale, fat tongue with a thin, white, moist coating

Pulse image: A deep, fine pulse in the cubit position

Treatment principles: Warm and supplement kidney yang

Rx: *Jin Gui Shen Qi Wan* (*Golden Cabinet* Kidney Qi Pills)

Ingredients:

prepared Radix Rehmanniae (*Shu Di*)
Fructus Corni Officinalis (*Shan Zhu Yu*)
Radix Dioscoreae Oppositae (*Shan Yao*)
Rhizoma Alismatis (*Ze Xie*)
Sclerotium Poriae Cocos (*Fu Ling*)

Cortex Radicis Moutan (*Dan Pi*)
Ramulus Cinnamomi (*Gui Zi*)
Radix Lateralis Praeparatus Aconiti Carmichaeli (*Fu Zi*)

Additions & subtractions: For cold feet, edema, tinnitus, deafness, dysuria, and low back pain, add Cornu Parvum Cervi (*Lu Rong*) and Fructus Schizandrae Chinensis (*Wu Wei Zi*). This results in *Shi Bu Wan* (Ten Supplements Pills). If cold is more severe, replace Ramulus Cinnamomi with Cortex Cinnamomi (*Rou Gui*). For nocturia, add Fructus Schizandrae Chinensis (*Wu Wei Zi*). For impotence, add Radix Morindae Officinalis (*Ba Ji Rou*), Herba Cistanchis (*Rou Cong Rong*), Herba Cynomorii Songarici (*Suo Yang*), and Fructus Lycii Chinensis (*Gou Qi Zi*).

Acupuncture & moxibustion: *Shen Shu* (Bl 23), *Guan Yuan* (CV 4), *Ming Men* (GV 4), *Fu Liu* (Ki 7), *San Yin Jiao* (Sp 6)

Auxiliary points: If there is dizziness, add *Bai Hui* (GV 20).

Key advice: Kidney yang vacuity may also present with a reddish tongue, a dry mouth, and flushed face. In this case, kidney yang has lost its root in its lower origin and is counterflowing upward. In that case, there will be cold feet below. Most often in clinical practice, kidney yang vacuity complicates other patterns, such as spleen/kidney yang vacuity and liver/kidney yang vacuity.

Kidney Vacuity, Water Spilling Over

Disease causes, disease mechanisms: Due to age or enduring disease, kidney yang vacuity may fail to transform and transport water, which then accumulates as water swelling.

Main symptoms: Low back and knee soreness and weakness, cold feet, severe edema, urinary strangury

Tongue & coating: A pale tongue with a thin, white, moist coating

Pulse image: Deep and fine

Treatment principles: Supplement the kidneys, warm yang, and seep water

Rx: *Ji Sheng Shen Qi Wan* (*Aid the Living* Kidney Qi Pills)

Ingredients:

prepared Radix Rehmanniae (*Shu Di*)
Fructus Corni Officinalis (*Shan Zhu Yu*)
Radix Dioscoreae Oppositae (*Shan Yao*)
Rhizoma Alismatis (*Ze Xie*)
Sclerotium Poriae Cocos (*Fu Ling*)
Cortex Radicis Moutan (*Dan Pi*)
Ramulus Cinnamomi (*Gui Zi*)
Radix Lateralis Praeparatus Aconiti Carmichaeli (*Fu Zi*)
Radix Cyathulae (*Chuan Niu Xi*)
Semen Plantaginis (*Che Qian Zi*)

Acupuncture & moxibustion: *Shen Shu* (Bl 23), *Pang Guang Shu* (Bl 28), *Shui Fen* (CV 9), *Shen Que* (CV 8), *Yin Ling Quan* (Sp 9)

Key advice: This pattern is also described in the chapter on fluids and humors pattern discrimination under the heading phlegm rheum.

Kidney Water Insulting the Heart

Disease causes, disease mechanisms: Due to age or enduring disease, kidney yang vacuity may fail to transport and transform water, which first accumulates and then counterflows upward, affecting the function of the heart.

Main symptoms: Low back and knee soreness and weakness, lack of warmth in the four limbs, edema, urinary strangury, heart palpitations, shortness of breath, chest pain, cyanotic lips and nails

Tongue & coating: A dark, purplish tongue with a thin, white, moist coating

Pulse image: A bound or regularly intermittent pulse

Treatment principles: Emergency supplement the kidneys and warm yang

Rx: *Si Wei Hui Yang Yin* (Four Flavors Rescue Yang Drink)

Ingredients:

Radix Panacis Ginseng (*Ren Shen*)
Radix Lateralis Praeparatus Aconiti Carmichaeli (*Fu Zi*)
blast-fried Rhizoma Zingiberis Officinalis (*Pao Jiang*)
Radix Glycyrrhizae (*Gan Cao*)

Acupuncture & moxibustion: *Shen Shu* (Bl 23), *Ming Men* (GV 4), *Xin Shu* (Bl 15), *Nei Guan* (Per 6), *Zu San Li* (St 36), *Shui Fen* (CV 9)

Key advice: This is an emergency condition that requires prompt treatment. The patient should also be referred to a Western physician for diagnosis and follow-up.

Kidney Yin Vacuity

Disease causes, disease mechanisms: This pattern is mainly due to insufficient natural endowment, aging, and enduring disease. However, it may also be due to excess sex, prolonged overtaxation, prolonged emotional stress, the sequelae of a warm disease, and excessive blood loss.

Main symptoms: Low back soreness and weakness, loose teeth, loss of hair, tinnitus or deafness, dizziness, low-grade afternoon fever, tidal fever, malar flushing, spermatorrhea or premature ejaculation, early menstruation, uterine bleeding, amenorrhea

Tongue & coating: A red tongue with a thin, yellow, scanty, dry, or absent coating

Pulse image: A deep, fine, rapid pulse

Treatment principles: Supplement the kidneys and enrich yin

Rx: *Liu Wei Di Huang Wan* (Six Flavors Rehmannia Pills)

Ingredients:

prepared Radix Rehmanniae (*Shu Di*)
Radix Dioscoreae Oppositae (*Shan Yao*)
Fructus Corni Officinalis (*Shan Zhu Yu*)
Sclerotium Poriae Cocos (*Fu Ling*)

Rhizoma Alismatis (*Ze Xie*)
Cortex Radicis Moutan (*Mu Dan Pi*)

Acupuncture & moxibustion: *Shen Shu* (Bl 23), *Yin Gu* (Ki 10), *Tai Xi* (Ki 3), *San Yin Jiao* (Sp 6), *Guan Yuan* (CV 4)

Auxiliary points: Add local points for local problems.

Key advice: The above guiding formula is the most famous one for kidney yin vacuity. However, kidney yin vacuity complicates a number of other patterns, such as liver/kidney vacuity, liver/kidney yin and yang vacuity, (spleen) qi and (kidney) yin vacuity, lung/kidney yin vacuity, and heart/kidney yin vacuity.

Yin Vacuity, Effulgent Fire

Disease causes, disease mechanisms: This pattern may be due to constitutional insufficiency, age, enduring disease, overtaxation, or excessive sex. Yin is insufficient to control yang; so fire counterflows upward.

Main symptoms: Night sweats, tidal fever, heat in the five hearts, spermatorrhea, premature ejaculation, increased sexual libido, heart palpitations, malar flush, dizziness, tinnitus, polyuria with scant, yellow urine, red lips, possible dry throat and cough

Tongue & coating: A red tongue with scanty, yellow coating

Pulse image: A fine, rapid or slippery, rapid, floating, surging pulse, especially in the inch positions

Treatment principles: Supplement the kidneys, enrich yin, and drain fire

Rx: *Zhi Bai Di Huang Wan* (Anemarrhena & Phellodendron Rehmannia Pills)

Ingredients:

Rhizoma Anemarrhenae (*Zhi Mu*)
Cortex Phellodendri (*Huang Bai*)
prepared Radix Rehmanniae (*Shu Di*)
Radix Dioscoreae Oppositae (*Shan Yao*)

Fructus Corni Officinalis (*Shan Zhu Yu*)
Sclerotium Poriae Cocos (*Fu Ling*)
Rhizoma Alismatis (*Ze Xie*)
Cortex Radicis Moutan (*Mu Dan Pi*)

Acupuncture & moxibustion: *Shen Shu* (Bl 23), *Yin Quan* (Ki 10), *Tai Xi* (Ki 3), *San Yin Jiao* (Sp 6), *Guan Yuan* (CV 4)

Auxiliary points: If there are night sweats, add *Xin Xi* (Ht 6) and *Hou Xi* (SI 3).

Key advice: This pattern is a commonly seen one in clinical practice. The difference between it and the preceding pattern are that there are more symptoms of heat counterflowing upward in this pattern.

Kidney Essence Insufficiency

Disease causes, disease mechanisms: Kidney essence insufficiency may be either due to former heaven (*i.e.*, prenatal) or latter heaven (*i.e.*, postnatal) causes. Former heaven causes are inherited at the moment of conception. Latter heaven causes include excessive sex, severe, acute, or enduring fear or fright, aging, enduring illness, or overtaxation. In terms of fear and fright, these may damage the kidney qi, which then fails to astringe and secure the essence in the form of the stools, menstrual blood, urination, or reproductive essence.

Main symptoms: Childhood retardation in standing, walking, hair growth, development of teeth and speech, delayed closure of the fontanel, lack of muscle strength, senile dementia, mental dullness, poor memory, lassitude, dizziness, deafness and tinnitus, amenorrhea, infertility, premature graying or loss of hair

Tongue & coating: Variable

Pulse image: Deep and weak or possibly choppy

Treatment principles: Supplement the kidneys and fill the essence

Rx: *Bu Shen Di Huang Wan* (Supplement the Kidneys Rehmannia Pills)

Ingredients:

Cornu Parvum Cervi (*Lu Rong*)
Radix Achyranthis Bidentatae (*Niu Xi*)
prepared Radix Rehmanniae (*Shu Di Huang*)
Fructus Corni Officinalis (*Shan Zhu Yu*)
dry Radix Dioscoreae Oppositae (*Gan Shan Yao*)
Rhizoma Alismatis (*Ze Xie*)
Sclerotium Poriae Cocos (*Fu Ling*)
Cortex Radicis Moutan (*Dan Pi*)

Acupuncture & moxibustion: *Shen Shu* (Bl 23), *Zhi Shi* (Bl 47), *Guan Yuan* (CV 4), *Da Zhong* (Ki 4), *San Yin Jiao* (Sp 6), *Zu San Li* (St 36)

Key advice: Essence is supplemented most directly by what the Chinese call bloody medicinals. These are medicinals made from animal tissue, such as the Pilose Deer Antler above. This pattern is seen either in children, in the elderly, or in those who have prematurely squandered their essence through excessive sex and use of so-called recreational drugs.

True Yin on the Verge of Exhaustion

Disease causes, disease mechanisms: Due to external invasion, liver/kidney yin may become damaged. This, in turn, results in the arising of vacuity heat, which may lead to the stirring of internal wind.

Main symptoms: Lassitude, deafness, a dry throat, black, sooty teeth, heat in the palms of the hands and soles of the feet

Tongue & coating: A dry, dark red tongue

Pulse image: A vacuous or rapid, irregularly interrupted pulse

Treatment principles: Nourish yin and extinguish the wind

Rx: *Da Ding Feng Zhu* (Great Stabilize Wind Pearls)

Ingredients:

Chicken Egg Yolk (*Ji Zi Huang*)
Gelatinum Corii Asini (*E Jiao*)
Radix Albus Paeoniae Lactiflorae (*Bai Shao*)
mix-fried Radix Glycyrrhizae (*Zhi Gan Cao*)
Fructus Schisandrae Chinensis (*Wu Wei Zi*)
uncooked Radix Rehmanniae (*Sheng Di*)
Tuber Ophiopogonis Japonicae (*Mai Men Dong*)
Semen Cannabis Sativae (*Huo Ma Ren*)
Plastrum Testudinis (*Gui Ban*)
Carapax Amydae Sinensis (*Bie Jia*)
Concha Ostreae (*Mu Li*)

Additions & subtractions: If there is wheezing and dyspnea due to concomitant qi vacuity, add Radix Panacis Ginseng (*Ren Shen*). If there is spontaneous sweating also due to qi vacuity, add Os Draconis (*Long Gu*), Radix Panacis Ginseng (*Ren Shen*), and Semen Levis Tritici (*Fu Xiao Mai*). For lingering low-grade fever, add Radix Cynanchi (*Bai Wei*) and Cortex Radicis Lycii Chinensis (*Di Gu Pi*).

Acupuncture & moxibustion: *San Yin Jiao* (Sp 6), *Tai Xi* (Ki 3), *Yin Xi* (Ht 6), *Zu San Li* (St 36), *Shen Shu* (Bl 23)

Key advice: According to triple burner pattern discrimination, this is a lower burner pattern. True yin is another name for kidney yin.

Heat Burning True Yin

Disease causes, disease mechanisms: If heat evils endure internally for a long time without healing, such internal heat may consume and damage yin fluids. Eventually this damages kidney yin, giving rise to yin vacuity, vacuity heat signs and symptoms.

Main symptoms: Low fever, a red facial complexion, heat in palms of the hands and soles of the feet, dry teeth and mouth, deafness

Tongue & coating: A dry, thin, dark red tongue without coating

Pulse image: A vacuous, rapid, vacuous, large, or fine, rapid pulse

Treatment principles: Nourish yin and engender fluids

Rx: *Jia Jian Fu Mai Tang* (Modified Restore the Pulse Decoction)

Ingredients:

mix-fried Radix Glycyrrhizae (*Zhi Gan Cao*)
uncooked Radix Rehmanniae (*Sheng Di*)
Radix Albus Paeoniae Lactiflorae (*Bai Shao*)
Tuber Ophiopogonis Japonicae (*Mai Men Dong*)
Gelatinum Corii Asini (*E Jiao*)
Semen Cannabis Sativae (*Huo Ma Ren*)

Acupuncture & moxibustion: *Shen Shu* (Bl 23), *Tai Xi* (Ki 3), *Fu Liu* (Ki 7), *Yong Quan* (Ki 1), *Gan Shu* (Bl 18)

Key advice: This pattern specifically describes yin vacuity due to lingering heat evils. According to triple burner pattern discrimination, this is also a lower burner pattern.

Cold Dampness Damaging the Kidneys

Disease causes, disease mechanisms: Cold damp evils may damage the *shao yin*, thus affecting kidney yang and giving rise to signs and symptoms associated with the kidneys.

Main symptoms: Scanty urine, edema, especially in lower body, pitting edema, low back soreness, cold limbs, aversion to cold

Tongue & coating: A tender, pale tongue with a white, slimy coating

Pulse image: A deep, fine, or wiry pulse

Treatment principles: Warm yang and disinhibit urination

Rx: *Zhen Wu Tang* (True Warrior Decoction)

Ingredients:

Radix Lateralis Praeparatus Aconiti Carmichaeli (*Fu Zi*)

Rhizoma Atractylodis Macrocephalae (*Bai Zhu*)
Sclerotium Poriae Cocos (*Fu Ling*)
uncooked Rhizoma Zingiberis (*Sheng Jiang*)
Radix Albus Paeoniae Lactiflorae (*Bai Shao*)

Additions & subtractions: If spleen vacuity is prominent with diarrhea, remove the Peony and add dry Rhizoma Zingiberis (*Gan Jiang*). If there is coughing, add Fructus Schizandrae Chinensis (*Wu Wei Zi*), Herba Cum Radice Asari (*Xi Xin*), and dry Rhizoma Zingiberis (*Gan Jiang*). If there is polyuria, remove the Poria. If there is unstoppable spontaneous perspiration, add Radix Panacis Ginseng (*Ren Shen*), Radix Astragali Membranacei (*Huang Qi*), and Fructus Schizandrae Chinensis (*Wu Wei Zi*). For vomiting due to water stagnation in the stomach, subtract Aconite and increase the dosage of uncooked Ginger.

Acupuncture & moxibustion: *Shen Shu* (Bl 23), *Qi Hai* (CV 6), *Shui Fen* (CV 9), *San Yin Jiao* (Sp 6), *Yin Ling Quan* (Sp 9), *Pi Shu* (Bl 20)

Key advice: This pattern is categorized by triple burner pattern discrimination as another lower burner pattern. Its signs and symptoms are all spleen/kidney yang vacuity symptoms due to damage by damp cold evils in the *shao yin* aspect. This pattern is often encountered in patients at the end stages of serious, life-threatening diseases, such as AIDS, liver cirrhosis, and heart failure.

Kidney Qi Migratory Wind

Disease causes, disease mechanisms: If internally kidney qi is smoldering and externally there is contraction of wind evils, then evils may become depressed and steam the skin and muscles, thus giving rise to this condition.

Main symptoms: Red, swollen lower legs and feet, in form like a cloud, migratory burning and pain

Tongue & coating: A red tongue

Pulse image: A floating, rapid pulse

Treatment principles: Clear heat and course wind, drain fire and resolve toxins

Rx: *Shuang Jie Tong Sheng San* (Doubly Resolving, Communicating with the Sages Powder)

Ingredients:

Gypsum Fibrosum (*Shi Gao*)
Radix Glycyrrhizae (*Gan Cao*)
Radix Ledebouriellae Sesloidis (*Fang Feng*)
Radix Ligustici Wallichii (*Chuan Xiong*)
Radix Angelicae Sinensis (*Dang Gui*)
Radix Albus Paeoniae Lactiflorae (*Bai Shao*)
Radix Et Rhizoma Rhei (*Da Huang*)
Herba Menthae Haplocalycis (*Bo He*)
Herba Ephedrae (*Ma Huang*)
Talcum (*Hua Shi*)
Radix Scutellariae Baicalensis (*Huang Qin*)
Radix Platycodi Grandiflori (*Jie Geng*)
Herba Schizonepetae Tenuifoliae (*Jing Jie*)
Rhizoma Atractylodis Macrocephalae (*Bai Zhu*)
Fructus Gardeniae Jasminoidis (*Zhi Zi*)
Semen Praeparatus Sojae (*Dan Dou Chi*)
Bulbus Allii Fistulosi (*Cong Bai*)

Key advice: This condition is also called lower leg cinnabar toxins. It is usually categorized as an external medicine condition or pattern.

Urinary Bladder Damp Heat

Disease causes, disease mechanisms: This pattern is due to invasion by external damp heat evils or to dampness pouring downward from the middle burner. Most commonly in Westerners, it is caused and aggravated by overeating sugars and sweets. Thus dampness is engendered in the spleen, which percolates downward to the lower burner. This dampness then obstructs the free flow of yang qi in the lower burner and transforms into damp heat. Such transformation into heat is even more likely and is facilitated by liver depression transforming into heat.

Main symptoms: Hot strangury, bloody strangury, if dampness is more severe, turbid urination, if heat is more severe, red urination, astringent and painful urination, dribbling and dripping, if severe, complete urinary blockage, lower abdominal tension and fullness, a dry mouth

Tongue & coating: A dry tongue with a slimy, yellow tongue coating

Pulse image: A slippery, rapid pulse

Treatment principles: Clear heat and drain fire, disinhibit water and free strangury

Rx: *Ba Zheng San* (Eight Correcting [Ingredients] Powder)

Ingredients:

Semen Plantaginis (*Che Qian Zi*)
Herba Dianthi (*Qu Mai*)
Herba Polygoni Avicularis (*Bian Xu*)
Talcum (*Hua Shi*)
Fructus Gardeniae Jasminoidis (*Shan Zhi Zi Ren*)
Radix Glycyrrhizae (*Gan Cao*)
Caulis Akebiae (*Mu Tong*)
Radix Et Rhizoma Rhei (*Da Huang*)
Medulla Junci Effusi (*Deng Xin Cao*)

Additions & subtractions: For bloody urine, add Rhizoma Imperatae Cylindricae (*Bai Mao Gen*), Herba Cephalanoplos (*Xiao Ji*), and Herba Ecliptae Prostratae (*Han Lian Cao*). For stones in the urinary tract, add Spora Lygodii (*Hai Jin Sha*), Herba Desmodii (*Jin Qian Cao*), and Endothelium Corneum Gigeriae Galli (*Ji Nei Jin*). For turbid urination, add Rhizoma Dioscoreae Hypoglaucae (*Bi Xie*) and Rhizoma Acori Graminei (*Shi Chang Pu*). For urinary retention, increase the dosage of Talcum, Polygonum Avicularis, and Akebia and add Cortex Phellodendri (*Huang Bai*) and Cortex Cinnamomi (*Rou Gui*).

Acupuncture & moxibustion: *Qu Quan* (Liv 8), *San Yin Jiao* (Sp 6), *Yin Ling Quan* (Sp 9), *Zhong Ji* (CV 3), *Pang Guang Shu* (Bl 28), *Ci Liao* (Bl 32)

Key advice: The above formula is for acute cystitis and acute prostatitis. Since most Westerners suffer from underlying spleen vacuity with dampness, this formula should not be used too long unmodified.

2
Yin & Yang Pattern Discrimination

Most yin and yang patterns, whether replete or vacuous, have already been described under viscera and bowel pattern discrimination. However, there are two yin yang patterns in particular that stand alone and are important to recognize. They are yang desertion and yin desertion. These patterns both describe emergency conditions requiring prompt and forceful treatment.

Yang Desertion

Disease causes, disease mechanisms: Yang desertion is due to any extreme detriment and damage to the yang qi. This is most often due to continuous, extreme vomiting, diarrhea, perspiration, or bleeding or other injury.

Main symptoms: Chills, cold skin, cold limbs, profuse cold and sticky sweating, absence of thirst, preference for hot drinks, feeble breathing, fatigued spirit, exhaustion

Tongue & coating: A pale tongue with a white, slimy coating

Pulse image: A deep, fine or deep, faint pulse

Treatment principles: Rescue yang and stem desertion

Rx: *Si Ni Tang* (Four Counterflows Decoction)

Ingredients:

Radix Lateralis Praeparatus Aconiti Carmichaeli (*Fu Zi*)
dry Rhizoma Zingiberis (*Gan Jiang*)
mix-fried Radix Glycyrrhizae (*Zhi Gan Cao*)

Acupuncture & moxibustion: *Guan Yuan* (CV 4), *Bai Hui* (GV 20), *Shen Que* (CV 8), *Zu San Li* (St 36),

Key advice: This pattern is an emergency condition requiring immediate and strong treatment. Be sure to keep the patient warm. If associated with shock, also elevate the feet.

Yin Desertion

Disease causes, disease mechanisms: This pattern is due to excessive sweating damaging both the qi and yin in turn due to summerheat stroke or heat stroke.

Main symptoms: Oily perspiration, a flushed red facial complexion and red lips, hot skin, warm hands and feet, thirst and preference for cold drinks, restlessness, shortness of breath and rapid breathing, aversion to heat

Tongue & coating: A pale red tongue with a thin, dry coating

Pulse image: A fine, weak, rapid pulse

Treatment principles: Nourish qi and yin

Rx: *Sheng Mai San* (Engender the Pulse Powder)

Ingredients:

Radix Panacis Ginseng (*Ren Shen*)
Tuber Ophiopogonis Japonicae (*Mai Men Dong*)
Fructus Schisandrae Chinensis (*Wu Wei Zi*)

Additions & subtractions: For excessive sweating with reddish yellow, scanty, astringent urination, add Radix Astragali Membranacei (*Huang Qi*) and Radix Angelicae Sinensis (*Dang Gui*). Because this is a yin vacuity pattern, is important not to use medicinals that seep dampness as these would only damage yin even more. If heart palpitations are marked, add Ramulus Cinnamomi (*Gui Zhi*), Concha Ostreae (*Mu Li*), and Os Draconis (*Long Gu*).

Acupuncture & moxibustion: *Tai Xi* (Ki 3), *Shui Gou* (GV 26), *Guan Yuan* (CV 4), *Yong Quan* (Ki 1), *Zu San Li* (St 36), *Nei Guan* (Per 6)

3
Qi & Blood Pattern Discrimination

Most qi and blood patterns have been discussed under viscera and bowel pattern discrimination. This is because, in clinical practice the qi represents the functioning of this or that particular viscus or bowel. Therefore, we have discussed liver depression, qi stagnation, heart qi vacuity, spleen qi vacuity, upward counterflow of lung qi, and so on. Likewise, we have discussed liver blood vacuity, heart blood vacuity, and heart blood stasis. However, there are several patterns pertaining to the qi and blood in general that are not discussed *vis à vis* the viscera and bowels.

Qi Desertion

Disease causes, disease mechanisms: This pattern is due to extreme fatigue, enduring disease, or any other cause that results in great vacuity of the qi. The qi, being so weak and deficient, can then not restrain and contain the body fluids, which exit profusely.

Main symptoms: Abrupt onset, profuse cold sweating, feeble breathing, urinary incontinence, a pale facial complexion, desire for hot drinks, cold skin, cold limbs, aversion to cold, and, in extreme cases, loss of consciousness

Tongue & coating: A pale tongue with a white coating

Pulse image: A deep, faint, or absent pulse

Treatment principles: Greatly supplement the qi, return yang and stem desertion

Rx: *Si Wei Hui Yang Yin* (Four Flavors Return Yang Drink)

Ingredients:

Radix Panacis Ginseng (*Ren Shen*)
Radix Lateralis Praeparatus Aconiti Carmichaeli (*Fu Zi*)

blast-fried Rhizoma Zingiberis (*Pao Jiang*)
Radix Glycyrrhizae (*Gan Cao*)

Acupuncture & moxibustion: *Ren Zhong* (GV 26), *Bai Hui* (GV 20), *Su Liao* (GV 25), *Shen Que* (CV 8)

Key advice: This pattern is essentially the same as yang desertion above. It is an emergency condition requiring strong, speedy treatment.

Sinking of the Great Qi

Disease causes, disease mechanisms: The great or *da qi* referred to in the name of this pattern is synonymous with the ancestral, or *zong qi*. This is the qi that gathers in the chest and is responsible for both the functioning of the lungs and the functioning of the heart. This qi is, therefore, consumed by the functioning of both these viscera. If these viscera consume more of this *da qi* than can be supplied by the spleen and stomach, it becomes vacuous and sinks, therefore failing to carry out its functions. In addition, this sinking results in the inhibited flow of qi and blood. Vacuity of this *da* or *zong qi* may be due to overtaxation, internal damage by the seven affects, enduring diseases of the lungs and/or heart, and spleen disease failing to upbear and thus provide nourishment to the heart and lungs.

Main symptoms: Dyspnea, an empty sensation in the chest, a downbearing sensation in the lower abdomen, easy anger, possible alternating heat and cold, edema, fullness in the chest, fatigue, dry throat, frequent yawning

Tongue & coating: A fat tongue with indentations of the teeth on the edges of the tongue and a thin, white coating. If there is stasis and stagnation, there may be a dark or purplish tongue.

Pulse image: A slow, deep, faint pulse especially in the inch positions on both hands or a choppy pulse in all six positions.

Treatment principles: Boost the qi and upbear the sunken

Rx: *Sheng Xian Tang* (Upbear the Sunken Decoction)

Ingredients:

Radix Astragali Membranacei (*Huang Qi*)
Rhizoma Anemarrhenae (*Zhi Mu*)
Radix Bupleuri (*Chai Hu*)
Rhizoma Cimicifugae (*Sheng Ma*)
Radix Platycodi Grandiflori (*Jie Geng*)

Acupuncture & moxibustion: *Shan Zhong* (CV 17), *Nei Guan* (Per 6), *Zu San Li* (St 36), *Fei Shu* (Bl 13), *Xin Shu* (Bl 15)

Key advice: This pattern is based on the insights of Zhang Xi-chun. It could be seen as a variation of downward sinking of central qi. However, the majority of its symptoms refer to the heart and lungs and not the spleen and stomach. According to Zhang Xi-chun, downward sinking of the central qi is a less serious pattern than sinking of the great qi. Nevertheless, long-term sinking of the central qi may lead to sinking of the great qi. Sinking of the great qi may be a life-threatening condition since it adversely affects the circulation of both the qi and blood.

Sinking of the Great Qi with Yang Vacuity of the Heart & Lungs

Disease causes, disease mechanisms: If the great qi is extremely vacuous and weak, heart and lung yang may also be vacuous and deficient, thus giving rise to signs and symptoms of cold.

Main symptoms: The above signs and symptoms of sinking of great qi plus coldness of the chest, upper back stiffness, aversion to cold, and dyspnea

Tongue & coating: A moist, pale blue or purplish tongue, fat tongue

Pulse image: Deep, faint, and slow, possibly regularly interrupted

Treatment principles: Boost the qi and upbear the sunken, warm yang and open the channels

Rx: *Hui Yang Sheng Xian Tang* (Rescue Yang & Upbear the Sunken Decoction)

Ingredients:

Radix Astragali Membranacei (*Huang Qi*)
dry Rhizoma Zingiberis (*Gan Jiang*)
Radix Angelicae Sinensis (*Dang Gui*)
Ramulus Cinnamomi (*Gui Zhi*)
Radix Glycyrrhizae (*Gan Cao*)

Acupuncture & moxibustion: Same as above but with moxibustion

Key advice: This is a potentially life-threatening condition and patients with this pattern should be monitored by a Western medical physician.

Sinking of the Great Qi with Qi Stagnation & Blood Stasis

Disease causes, disease mechanisms: If, due to the above-described causes and mechanisms, the great qi sinks downward, this may depress the qi. If the qi fails to flow freely and smoothly, the blood will also become inhibited. This is because the qi moves the blood and if the qi stops, the blood will stop.

Main symptoms: The above symptoms of sunken great qi plus body pain, lateral costal fullness and distention

Tongue & coating: A similar tongue to sunken great qi but possibly dark if there is qi depression or purplish or static spots or macules if there is blood stasis

Pulse image: A deep, faint, wiry or choppy pulse

Treatment principles: Boost the qi and upbear the sunken, regulate the qi and resolve depression, quicken the blood and open the network vessels

Rx: *Li Yu Sheng Xian Tang* (Regulate Depression & Upbear the Sunken Decoction)

Ingredients:

Radix Astragali Membranacei (*Huang Qi*)
Rhizoma Anemarrhenae (*Zhi Mu*)
Radix Bupleuri (*Chai Hu*)

Radix Angelicae Sinensis (*Dang Gui*)
Ramulus Cinnamomi (*Gui Zhi*)
Resina Myrrhae (*Mo Yao*)
Resina Olibani (*Ru Xiang*)

Acupuncture & moxibustion: The same as for sinking of great qi above plus *Tai Zhong* (Liv 4) and *He Gu* (LI 4)

Key advice: This pattern may also be evidence of a life-threatening pattern. Therefore, patients with this pattern should receive a Western medical diagnosis if there is any question about their condition. However, this pattern may also simply be a non-organic, stress-related reaction. If this pattern combines with one immediately above, it can be serious. Originally, sinking of great qi was associated with sudden death in otherwise seemingly healthy individuals.

Blood Vacuity

Disease causes, disease mechanisms: This pattern may be due to either the liver not treasuring the blood, traumatic injury resulting in bleeding, or either the heart, spleen, or kidneys not transforming and engendering the blood.

Main symptoms: Dizziness, tinnitus, heart palpitations, loss of sleep, blurred vision, a lusterless facial complexion and nails, generalized muscular tension, irregular menstruation with scanty flow, possible amenorrhea, occasional aching and pain, restless fetus during pregnancy, downward precipitation of blood that will not stop, postpartum lochia that will not stop, lower abdominal sagging pain, occasional fever and chills

Tongue & coating: A pale tongue

Pulse image: A wiry, fine or fine, choppy pulse

Treatment principles: Nourish and regulate the blood

Rx: *Si Wu Tang* (Four Materials Decoction)

Ingredients:

Radix Angelicae Sinensis (*Dang Gui*)
Radix Ligustici Wallichii (*Chuan Xiong*)

Radix Albus Paeoniae Lactiflorae (*Bai Shao*)
prepared dry Radix Rehmanniae (*Shu Gan Di Huang*)

Additions & subtractions: For anemia and heart palpitations, add Cortex Cinnamomi (*Rou Gui*), Sclerotium Poriae Cocos (*Fu Ling*), Rhizoma Atractylodis Macrocephalae (*Bai Zhu*), and Radix Glycyrrhizae (*Gan Cao*). This results in *Lian Zhu Yin* (Lotus & Pearl Drink).

Acupuncture & moxibustion: *Zu San Li* (St 36), *San Yin Jiao* (Sp 6), *Ge Shu* (Bl 17), *Gan Shu* (Bl 18), *Shen Shu* (Bl 23)

Key advice: In clinical practice, this pattern is rarely used. This is because blood vacuity is usually described as either qi *and* blood vacuity, as in the above modification for anemia and heart palpitations, or is further described as heart blood vacuity or liver blood vacuity. Blood vacuity may also complicate many other patterns. When blood vacuity does complicate other patterns, usually Dang Gui and prepared Rehmannia are added to other guiding formulas.

Blood Desertion

Disease causes, disease mechanisms: Blood desertion describes one's condition after having lost a large amount of blood. The reasons for such blood loss are many, including various types of heat and traumatic injury.

Main symptoms: A sallow yellow or somber white facial complexion, pale lips, tremor of the limbs, dark circles under the eyes, cold limbs, excessive cold sweating, feeble breath, and, in severe cases, loss of consciousness

Tongue & coating: A pale tongue

Pulse image: A fine, rapid vacuous pulse

Treatment principles: Supplement the qi and stem desertion

Rx: *Du Shen Tang* (Solitary Ginseng Decoction)

Ingredients:

Radix Panacis Ginseng (*Ren Shen*)

Additions & subtractions: For cold limbs, add Radix Lateralis Praeparatus Aconiti Carmichaeli (*Fu Zi*). For profuse sweating, add Os Draconis (*Long Gu*) and Concha Ostreae (*Mu Li*).

Acupuncture & moxibustion: *Ren Zhong* (GV 26), *Guan Yuan* (CV 4), *Qi Hai* (CV 6), *Bai Hui* (GV 20)

Key advice: The signs and symptoms within this pattern are mixed. There are the signs of blood vacuity, such as the pale or sallow facial complexion, lips, and nails. There are also signs and symptoms of qi vacuity, like the cold sweating and feeble breath. When blood is lost, the qi follows blood desertion. In order to stem such qi or yang desertion and because qi is the commander of the blood, Ginseng is given instead of blood-nourishing ingredients. Ginseng will stem further qi and/or blood desertion at the same time as promoting the transformation and engenderment of new blood. This is an emergency condition that requires speedy, forceful treatment.

Blood Stasis

Disease causes, disease mechanisms: Blood stasis may be due to qi stagnation failing to move the blood. It may be due to traumatic injury, including surgical injury, severing the channels and network vessels. In that case, blood flows outside the channels where it impedes the flow of subsequent qi, blood, and body fluids. Blood stasis may be hypothetically due to food stagnation impeding the qi, which then fails to move the blood. But it is more likely to be due to damp and or phlegm depression, in which case the mechanisms are basically the same. In addition, blood stasis may be due to either or both qi and blood vacuity. If qi is insufficient to move the blood, the blood will stop and become static, whereas if the blood is insufficient, it will fail to fill the vessels and thus maintain its free and smooth flow.

Main symptoms: In general, the symptoms of blood stasis are intense, fixed, piercing pain, concretions and conglomerations, accumulations and gatherings, bleeding, a dark facial complexion, dry, scaly, itchy skin, possible low-grade fever, visible congested, tortuous, purplish veins, hematomas, yellowish brown or grayish-blue maculae, a.k.a. liver or age spots

Tongue & coating: A dark red or purplish tongue with static spots or macules on the tongue

Pulse image: A fine, wiry, choppy pulse or even an irregular pulse

Treatment principles: Quicken the blood and dispel stasis

Rx: *Tao Hong Si Wu Tang* (Persica & Carthamus Four Materials Decoction)

Ingredients:

Semen Pruni Persicae (Tao Ren)
Flos Carthami Tinctorii (*Hong Hua*)
Radix Angelicae Sinensis (*Dang Gui*)
Radix Ligustici Wallichii (*Chuan Xiong*)
Radix Albus Paeoniae Lactiflorae (*Bai Shao*)
prepared dry Radix Rehmanniae (*Shu Gan Di Huang*)

Additions & subtractions: To reinforce the quickening of the blood and transformation of stasis, replace prepared Rehmannia with uncooked Radix Rehmanniae (*Sheng Di*) and White Peony with Radix Rubrus Paeoniae Lactiflorae (*Chi Shao*).

Acupuncture & moxibustion: *Xue Hai* (Sp 10), *Ge Shu* (Bl 17), *Zu San Li* (St 36), *He Gu* (LI 4)

Auxiliary points: Add local points depending upon the affected area.

Key advice: This pattern is a very generalized one. There are different degrees of blood stasis requiring different degrees of attacking. For instance, transforming stasis is milder than dispelling stasis, while dispelling stasis is milder than breaking the blood. In addition, blood stasis may affect any area of the body. It also commonly complicates other patterns, such as heat and stasis, phlegm and stasis, qi vacuity and stasis, blood vacuity and stasis, and so on.

Stasis in the Channels & Network Vessels

Disease causes, disease mechanisms: Blood stasis may arise due to strike or fall that severs the channels and network vessels. Thus the blood does not return to the channels but rather pools outside the channels where it is retained and becomes static. Blood stasis in the channels and network vessels may also be due to the presence of an enduring evil qi, which blocks and obstructs the flow of qi and blood. And lastly, blood stasis in the channels and network vessels may be due to qi and/or blood vacuity. In that case, there is insufficient qi to move the blood or insufficient blood to fill the vessels in order to ensure free and smooth flow.

Main symptoms: Pain in the joints, numbness of the limbs, hemiplegia

Tongue & coating: A dark, purplish tongue or the presence of static spots or macules on the tongue

Pulse image: A fine and wiry or choppy pulse

Treatment principles: Quicken the blood and move the qi, dispel stasis and open the network vessels

Rx: *Shen Tong Zhu Yu Tang* (Body Pain Dispel Stasis Decoction)

Ingredients:

Radix Gentianae Macrophyllae (*Qin Jiao*)
Semen Pruni Persicae (*Tao Ren*)
Flos Carthami Tinctorii (*Hong Hua*)
Radix Angelicae Sinensis (*Dang Gui*)
Radix Ligustici Wallichii (*Chuan Xiong*)
Radix Et Rhizoma Notopterygii (*Qiang Huo*)
Resina Myrrhae (*Mo Yao*)
Rhizoma Cyperi Rotundi (*Xiang Fu*)
Radix Cyathulae (*Chuan Niu Xi*)
Lumbricus (*Di Long*)
Radix Glycyrrhizae (*Gan Cao*)

Additions & subtractions: If there are signs of dampness and heat, add Rhizoma Atractylodis (*Cang Zhu*) and Cortex Phellodendri (*Huang Bai*). If there is concomitant weakness and fatigue, add Radix Astragali Membranacei (*Huang Qi*). If there is low back pain, add Cortex Eucommiae Ulmoidis (*Du Zhong*) and Radix Morindae Officinalis (*Ba Ji Tian*).

Acupuncture & moxibustion: *Xue Hai* (Sp 10), *Ge Shu* (Bl 17), *He Gu* (LI 4), *Zu San Li* (St 36), plus points on the affected channels

Key advice: If there is blood stasis in the channels and network vessels, search the body for small, purplish red or purplish blue veins. Using a three-edged needle, prick these in order to bleed them. This can treat recalcitrant, stubborn pain due to stasis in the network channels and is called network channel puncture (*luo ci*).

Blood Stasis in the Chest

Disease causes, disease mechanisms: This pattern may be due to traumatic injury or to enduring stress causing liver depression and qi stagnation. The liver controls the spreading of qi through the chest region and intercostal spaces. If the qi stops, eventually the blood will stop and become static.

Main symptoms: Chest pain and lateral costal regions that is enduring and fixed in location and piercing in nature, possible enduring, incessant hiccup, a choking sensation when drinking, palpitations, insomnia, irritability, lack of constancy in joy and anger, evening tidal fever

Tongue & coating: A dark red or purplish tongue or the presence of static spots or macules on the tongue

Pulse image: A wiry, choppy pulse

Treatment principles: Quicken the blood and dispel stasis, rectify the qi and open the network vessels

Rx: *Xue Fu Zhu Yu Tang* (Blood Mansion Dispel Stasis Decoction)

Ingredients:

Semen Pruni Persicae (*Tao Ren*)
Flos Carthami Tinctorii (*Hong Hua*)
Radix Angelicae Sinensis (*Dang Gui*)
Radix Ligustici Wallichii (*Chuan Xiong*)
Radix Rubrus Paeoniae Lactiflorae (*Chi Shao*)
Radix Cyathulae (*Chuan Niu Xi*)

Radix Bupleuri (*Chai Hu*)
Radix Platycodi Grandiflori (*Jie Geng*)
Fructus Aurantii (*Zhi Ke*)
uncooked Radix Rehmanniae (*Sheng Di*)
Radix Glycyrrhizae (*Gan Cao*)

Additions & subtractions: For lateral costal pain, add Tuber Curcumae (*Yu Jin*) and Bulbus Allii (*Xie Bai*). For immovable concretions below the ribs or immobile accumulations in the abdomen, add Tuber Curcumae (*Yu Jin*) and Radix Salviae Miltiorrhizae (*Dan Shen*) and remove Platycodon. For coronary artery disease, increase the dosages of Carthamus and Ligusticum and add Radix Salviae Miltiorrhizae (*Dan Shen*).

Acupuncture & moxibustion: *Nei Guan* (Per 6), *Tai Chong* (Liv 3), *He Gu* (LI 4), *Xue Hai* (Sp 10), *Shan Zhong* (CV 17), *Xin Bao Shu* (Bl 14), *Xin Shu* (Bl 15), *Ge Shu* (Bl 17)

Key advice: This pattern is very similar to heart blood stasis described above. However, the above formula treats blood stasis within the chest regardless of the affected organ. Since the heart rules the blood and governs the vessels, any stasis within the chest may show some heart signs, even if they are mostly psycho-emotional.

Stasis Binding in the Upper Abdomen

Disease causes, disease mechanisms: Blood stasis binding in the epigastrium may be due to anger, stress, and frustration, causing liver depression, qi stagnation. If this endures, this will eventually engender blood stasis, since the qi moves the blood. If the qi moves, the blood will move. If the qi stops, the blood will stop and become static.

Main symptoms: Masses in abdomen or in the hypochondriac region with pressure pain, subcutaneous varicose veins on abdominal wall, visible abdominal masses when lying supine

Tongue & coating: A dark, purplish tongue

Pulse image: A deep, choppy pulse

Treatment principles: Quicken the blood and dispel stasis, break the blood and disperse swelling

Rx: *Ge Xia Zhu Yu Tang* (Below the Diaphragm Dispel Stasis Decoction)

Ingredients:

stir-fried Feces Trogopterori Seu Pteromi (*Wu Ling Zhi*)
Radix Angelicae Sinensis (*Dang Gui*)
Radix Ligustici Wallichii (*Chuan Xiong*)
Semen Pruni Persicae (*Tao Ren*)
Cortex Radicis Moutan (*Mu Dan Pi*)
Radix Rubrus Paeoniae Lactiflorae (*Chi Shao*)
Radix Linderae Strychnifoliae (*Wu Yao*)
Rhizoma Corydalis Yanhusuo (*Yan Hu Suo*)
Radix Glycyrrhizae (*Gan Cao*)
Rhizoma Cyperi Rotundi (*Xiang Fu*)
Flos Carthami Tinctorii (*Hong Hua*)
Fructus Aurantii (*Zhi Ke*)

Acupuncture & moxibustion: *Tai Chong* (Liv 3), *Nei Guan* (Per 6), *Xue Hai* (Sp 10), *Zhang Men* (Liv 13), *Zhong Wan* (CV 12), *Qi Hai* (CV 6), *Ge Shu* (Bl 17)

Key advice: Palpable lumps in the upper abdomen should be diagnosed and monitored by a Western physician. Lumps that are hard, fixed, and immovable are difficult to treat with Chinese medicine alone and may be life-threatening if left untreated.

Stasis Binding in the Lower Abdomen

Disease causes, disease mechanisms: This pattern is also due mostly to untreated, unsoothed liver qi depression in turn due to anger, frustration, and stress. When the qi stops, the blood stops and becomes static. However, it may also be due to iatrogenesis, such as treatment of acute pelvic inflammatory disease only with heat-clearing medicinals, *i.e.*, Western antibiotics, use of oral birth control pills or intrauterine devices, and the sequelae of fallopian tube and seminal vesical ligation as well as artificial abortions. In these cases, blood stasis is created directly through physical impediment or through surgery severing the channels and network vessels.

Main symptoms: Lower abdominal pain that is chronic, fixed, and piercing in nature, possible palpable lumps within the abdomen that refuse pressure, clots in a woman's menstruate, menstrual irregularity, painful menstruation, amenorrhea, and possible infertility

Tongue & coating: A dark red or purplish tongue or the presence of static spots or macules on the tongue

Pulse image: Wiry and fine or wiry and choppy

Treatment principles: Quicken the blood and dispel stasis, warm the menses (when used for the treatment of gynecological diseases) and stop pain

Rx: _Shao Fu Zhu Yu Tang_ (Lower Abdomen Dispel Stasis Decoction)

Ingredients:

stir-fried Fructus Foeniculi Vulgaris (_Xiao Hui Xiang_)
stir-fried dry Rhizoma Zingiberis (_Gan Jiang_)
Rhizoma Corydalis Yanhusuo (_Yan Hu Suo_)
Radix Angelicae Sinensis (_Dang Gui_)
Radix Ligustici Wallichii (_Chuan Xiong_)
Resina Myrrhae (_Mo Yao_)
Cortex Cinnamomi (_Guan Gui_)
Radix Rubrus Paeoniae Lactiflorae (_Chi Shao_)
Pollen Typhae (_Pu Huang_)
stir-fried Feces Trogopterori Seu Pteromi (_Wu Ling Zhi_)

Additions & subtractions: If there are no symptoms of cold, such as relief of pain on obtaining warmth or cold feet, remove the dry Ginger and Cinnamon and add more qi-moving or blood quickening ingredients as indicated following the patient's condition. If there is insidious, enduring lower abdominal pain, add Radix Codonopsis Pilosulae (_Dang Shen_), Gelatinum Corii Asini (_E Jiao_), and prepared Radix Rehmanniae (_Shu Di_). If there is abdominal pain during menstruation that dislikes pressure and excessive bleeding, delete dry Ginger and Cinnamon and add uncooked Rhizoma Zingiberis (_Sheng Jiang_). If there is severe menstrual pain, add Radix Auklandiae (_Mu Xiang_) and Radix Albus Paeoniae Lactiflorae (_Bai Shao_).

Acupuncture & moxibustion: _Tai Chong_ (Liv 3), _San Yin Jiao_ (Sp 6), _Xue Hai_ (Sp 10), _He Gu_ (LI 4), _Qi Hai_ (CV 6), _Zhong Ji_ (CV 3), _Da Chang Shu_ (Bl 25)

Auxiliary points: For ovarian cysts, add *Zi Gong* (M-CA-18) and *Gui Lai* (St 29). For constipation, add *Tian Shu* (St 25). For pain on the wings of the lower abdomen, add *Dai Mai* (GB 26), *Jing Men* (GB 25), and *Zu Lin Qi* (GB 41).

Key advice: This is a commonly seen pattern in gynecological diseases characterized by either intense pain or palpable lumps.

Blood Heat

Disease causes, disease mechanisms: Due to depressive heat in turn due to stress, replete heat due to overeating acrid, peppery, hot foods and fatty, fried foods or drinking too much alcohol, or vacuity heat in turn due to enduring disease, bedroom taxation, or bodily vacuity, evil heat may enter the blood and cause it to move recklessly outside its pathways. In this case, heat damages the blood network vessels and the blood spills outside its channels and vessels, causing various types of bleeding.

Main symptoms: Vomiting up blood, coughing up blood, nosebleed, bloody stools, and other such hemorrhagic conditions. Bleeding due to heat tends to be excessive and bright red in color.

Tongue & coating: A crimson tongue with possible prickles. If due to replete heat, there will usually be a slimy, yellow coating. If due to depressive heat, there will usually be a thin, yellow coating. And if due to vacuity heat, there will be a scanty, yellow coating or no coating.

Pulse image: If due to replete heat, a slippery, rapid pulse. If due to depressive heat, a wiry, rapid pulse. And if due to vacuity heat, a fine, rapid pulse

Treatment principles: Clear heat, cool the blood, and stop bleeding

Rx: *Xi Jiao Di Huang Tang Jia Jian* (Rhinoceros Horn & Rehmannia Decoction with Additions & Subtractions)

Ingredients:

Cornu Bubali (*Shui Niu Jiao*)
uncooked Radix Rehmannia (*Sheng Di*)
Radix Rubrus Paeoniae Lactiflorae (*Chi Shao*)
Cortex Radicis Moutan (*Mu Dan Pi*)

Additions & subtractions: For replete heat, add Rhizoma Coptidis Chinensis (*Huang Lian*) and Radix Scutellariae Baicalensis (*Huang Qin*). For depressive heat, add Fructus Gardeniae Jasminoidis (*Shan Zhi Zi*) and Radix Scutellariae Baicalensis (*Huang Qin*). For vacuity heat, add Tuber Ophiopogonis Japonicae (*Mai Dong*), Radix Scrophulariae Ningpoensis (*Xuan Shen*), and Cortex Phellodendri (*Huang Bai*). Then for hematemesis and epistaxis, add Cacumen Biotae Orientalis (*Ce Bai Ye*), Rhizoma Imperatae Cylindricae (*Bai Mao Gen*), and Herba Ecliptae Prostratae (*Han Lian Cao*). For hemafecia, add Radix Sanguisorbae (*Di Yu*) and Flos Immaturus Sophorae Japonicae (*Huai Hua*). For severe bleeding, add powdered Radix Pseudoginseng (*San Qi Fen*).

Acupuncture & moxibustion: *Qu Chi* (LI 11), *Wei Zhong* (Bl 40), *Xue Hai* (Sp 10). For replete heat add *Nei Ting* (St 44), *Zu San Li* (St 36), and *He Gu* (LI 4). For depressive heat, add *Qu Ze* (Per 3) and *Xing Jian* (Liv 2). For vacuity heat, add *San Yin Jiao* (Sp 6) and *Tai Xi* (Ki 3). Then add local points depending on the sight of bleeding.

Key advice: Bleeding is considered a branch symptom that requires primary treatment. Therefore, one should first stop the bleeding and then one can go back and figure out exactly why the bleeding has occurred and correct the root pattern. For instance, in the case of depressive heat, one must also course the liver and resolve depression, while for vacuity heat, one must enrich yin and downbear fire.

Blood Heat, Blood Stasis

Disease causes, disease mechanisms: This pattern is most often due to extreme heat or fire toxins entering the blood aspect. There, this heat stews the juices and causes congelation and blood stasis. Thus this pattern is mostly seen in acute infectious diseases that are characterized as *wen bing* or warm diseases and that are accompanied by high fever and erythema or purpuric rashes.

Main symptoms: Vexation and restlessness, various types of bleeding, possible erythema or purpuric rashes, fever that worsens at night, possible delirium

Tongue & coating: A dry, crimson tongue

Pulse image: A fine, rapid pulse

Treatment principles: Clear heat and resolve toxins, cool the blood and dispel stasis

Rx: *Qing Ying Tang Jia Jian* (Clear the Constructive Decoction with Additions & Subtractions)

Ingredients:

Cornu Bubali (*Shui Niu Jiao*)
Radix Scrophulariae Ningpoensis (*Xuan Shen*)
uncooked Radix Rehmanniae (*Sheng Di Huang*)
Tuber Ophiopogonis Japonicae (*Mai Men Dong*)
Flos Lonicerae Japonicae (*Jin Yin Hua*)
Fructus Forsythiae Suspensae (*Lian Qiao*)
Rhizoma Coptidis Chinensis (*Huang Lian*)
Herba Lophatheri Gracilis (*Dan Zhu Ye*)
Radix Salviae Miltiorrhizae (*Dan Shen*)

Additions & subtractions: If yin fluids have been severely depleted, add Radix Glehniae Littoralis (*Sha Shen*) and Fructus Lycii Chinensis (*Gou Qi Zi*). If there is pronounced qi aspect fire, add Gypsum Fibrosum (*Shi Gao*). If fire has engendered stirring of internal wind with tremors and spasms, add Ramulus Uncariae Cum Uncis (*Gou Teng*), Cornu Antelopis Saiga-tataricae (*Ling Yang Jiao*), and Lumbricus (*Di Long*).

Acupuncture & moxibustion: *Xue Hai* (Sp 10), *Qu Chi* (LI 11), *Zu San Li* (St 36), *Tai Xi* (Ki 3), *Wei Zhong* (Bl 40), *Nei Ting* (St 44)

4
Fluids & Humors Pattern Discrimination

When it comes to fluids and humors patterns, most of these and particularly the vacuity and insufficiency patterns are included under viscera and bowel pattern discrimination. For instance, stomach yin vacuity implies vacuity of stomach fluids. Fluids and humors *per se* are both types of righteous yin. However, when fluids accumulate pathologically, they may become either rheum evils or phlegm evils. Therefore, under the heading of fluids and humors pattern discrimination, we list below a number of rheum evil and phlegm evil patterns. Other dampness, rheum, and phlegm patterns are listed under viscera and bowel pattern discrimination.

Rheum Evils

Spillage Rheum

Disease causes, disease mechanisms: This pattern may be due to any cause damaging the spleen, whether internal, external, or neither internal nor external. In this case, water dampness spills over into the skin where it blocks and obstructs the flow of defensive qi, which then causes stagnation of the lung qi and loss of the lungs' diffusion and downbearing.

Main symptoms: Chills, no sweating, edema in the limbs, generalized aching, lassitude, no thirst, excessive, white, frothy phlegm, possible dyspnea

Tongue & coating: A white tongue coating

Pulse image: Floating and wiry or tight pulse

Treatment principles: Resolve the exterior and diffuse the lungs, downbear the qi and eliminate dampness

Rx: *Xiao Qing Long Tang* (Minor Blue-green Dragon Decoction)

Ingredients:

Herba Ephedrae (*Ma Huang*)
Ramulus Cinnamomi (*Gui Zhi*)
dry Rhizoma Zingiberis (*Gan Jiang*)
Herba Cum Radice Asari Sieboldi (*Xi Xin*)
Fructus Schisandrae Chinensis (*Wu Wei Zi*)
Radix Albus Paeoniae Lactiflorae (*Bai Shao*)
Rhizoma Pinelliae Ternatae (*Ban Xia*)
mix-fried Radix Glycyrrhizae (*Zhi Gan Cao*)

Additions & subtractions: For severe exterior cold, increase the dosages of Ephedra and Cinnamon. For excessive phlegm, inability to lie down, a wel, slimy tongue coating, and a wiry, tight or wire, slippery pulse, increase Asarum and Pinellia and add uncooked Rhizoma Zingiberis (*Sheng Jiang*). For pronounced nasal congestion, runny nose, and headache, change dry Ginger to uncooked Ginger and White Peony to Rubrus Paeoniae Lactiflorae (*Chi Shao*) and add Radix Ledebouriellae Sesloidis (*Fang Feng*) and Herba Schizonepetae Tenuifoliae (*Jing Jie*).

Acupuncture & moxibustion: *Fei Shu* (Bl 13), *He Gu* (LI 4), *Yin Ling Quan* (Sp 9), *Shui Fen* (CV 9), *Pian Li* (LI 6)

Key advice: This pattern is also called phlegm rheum in the limbs and is similar to wind water.

For patients with a stronger constitution and internal heat, *Da Qing Long Tang* (Great Blue-green Dragon Decoction) is indicated: Herba Ephedrae (*Ma Huang*), Semen Pruni Armeniacae (*Xing Ren*), Ramulus Cinnamomi (*Gui Zhi*), mix-fried Radix Glycyrrhizae (*Zhi Gan Cao*), Gypsum Fibrosum (*Shi Gao*), uncooked Rhizoma Zingiberis (*Sheng Jiang*), and Fructus Zizyphi Jujubae (*Da Zao*).

Propping Rheum

Disease causes, disease mechanisms: Damage to the spleen causes dampness and fluids to accumulate between the diaphragm and heart. This prevents the downbearing of the qi and may result in upward counterflow of either or both the lung and stomach qi.

Main symptoms: Dyspnea and cough, chest fullness and oppression, vomiting of phlegm, inability to lie down, swelling and distention of the body

Tongue & coating: A white, moist tongue coating

Pulse image: A wiry, replete pulse in the inch and bar positions

Treatment principles: Eliminate cold and evil fluids or drain the lungs and eliminate evil fluids

Rx: *Xiao Qing Long Tang Jia Wei* (Minor Blue-green Dragon Decoction with Added Flavors)

Ingredients:

Herba Ephedrae (*Ma Huang*)
Ramulus Cinnamomi (*Gui Zhi*)
dry Rhizoma Zingiberis (*Gan Jiang*)
Herba Cum Radice Asari Sieboldi (*Xi Xin*)
Fructus Schisandrae Chinensis (*Wu Wei Zi*)
Radix Albus Paeoniae Lactiflorae (*Bai Shao*)
Rhizoma Pinelliae Ternatae (*Ban Xia*)
Sclerotium Poriae Cocos (*Fu Ling*)
mix-fried Radix Glycyrrhizae (*Zhi Gan Cao*)

Additions & subtractions: If cough and dyspnea are severe, increase the dosage of Schizandra and reduce the amounts of dry Ginger and Asarum. If phlegm is difficult to expectorate, remove Peony and decrease the amount of Schizandra. If there is concomitant internal heat with cough, yellow phlegm, and a wiry, rapid pulse, add Gypsum Fibrosum (*Shi Gao*).

If propping rheum is complicated by an attack by external wind, there will be aversion to wind, cough, dyspnea, wheezing, and a floating pulse. In that case, use *She Gan Ma Huang Tang* (Belamcanda & Ephedra Decoction): Rhizoma Belamcandae Chinensis (*She Gan*), Herba Ephedrae (*Ma Huang*), Radix Asteris Tatarici (*Zi Wan*), Flos Tussilaginis Farfarae (*Kuan Dong Hua*), Rhizoma Pinelliae Ternatae (*Ban Xia*), Herba Cum Radice Asari Sieboldi (*Xi Xin*), Fructus Schizandrae Chinensis (*Wu Wei Zi*), uncooked Rhizoma Zingiberis (*Sheng Jiang*), and Fructus Zizyphi Jujubae (*Da Zao*).

If propping rheum has endured for a long time and has damaged the lungs, spleen, and kidneys, there will be cough, dyspnea with inability to lie down, thick, white phlegm, fear of cold, lower and upper back pain, an edema, especially of the face and lower limbs, a white tongue coating, and a fine, wiry or tight pulse due to cold rheum with yang qi vacuity. In that case use *Gui Ling Wu Wei Gan Cao Tang Jia Wei* (Cinnamon, Poria, Schizandra & Licorice Decoction with Added Flavors): Ramulus Cinnamomi (*Gui Zhi*), Sclerotium Poriae Cocos (*Fu Ling*), Fructus Schizandrae Chinensis (*Wu Wei Zi*), Radix Glycyrrhizae (*Gan Cao*), Herba Cum Radice Asari Sieboldi (*Xi Xin*).

Acupuncture & moxibustion: *Ge Shu* (Bl 17), *Zhong Wan* (CV 12), *Xuan Ji* (CV 21), *Zhang Men* (Liv 13), *Shui Dao* (St 28), *Yin Ling Quan* (Sp 9)

Auxiliary points: If there is dyspnea and coughing, add *Ding Chuan* (M-BW-1b).

Key advice: This pattern is also called phlegm rheum above the diaphragm.

Suspended Rheum

Disease causes, disease mechanisms: This pattern is due to failure of the lungs to downbear and diffuse fluids and of the spleen to transport and a transform water, which then accumulates in the chest and lateral costal regions. If it counterflows upward, it may cause cough and shortness of breath.

Main symptoms: Cough causing pain in the chest and lateral costal regions, hard glomus beneath the heart, dry heaves and shortness of breath, headache, vertigo, possible chest pain extending to the upper back with the pain making breathing difficult

Tongue & coating: A white tongue coating

Pulse image: A deep, wiry pulse

Treatment principles: Attack and drive out water rheum

Rx: *Shi Zao Tang* (Ten Dates Decoction)

Ingredients:

Radix Euphorbiae Kansui (*Gan Sui*)

Radix Euphorbiae Seu Knoxiae (*Da Ji*)
Flos Daphnis Genkwae (*Yuan Hua*)

Acupuncture & moxibustion: *Zhang Men* (Liv 13), *Chi Ze* (Lu 5), *Zhong Wan* (CV 12), *Hua Rou Men* (St 24), *Shui Dao* (St 28)

Key advice: This pattern is also called phlegm rheum in the lateral costal region.

Because *Shi Zao Tang* is a strong attacking and precipitating formula, one should take care in its use. First, there should be no lingering evils in the exterior. Secondly, the patient should have a strong bodily constitution. Administer this decoction only once and wait for several days for it to take effect before administering it again. If there is mixed repletion and vacuity, administer supplements along with precipitation in order to dispel evils at the same time as harmonizing the righteous. If this prescription results in severe and continuous diarrhea, administer cold rice porridge in order to stop it.

Phlegm Rheum

Disease causes, disease mechanisms: Due to overtaxation, lack of discipline in eating and drinking, or excessive thinking, worry, and anxiety, the spleen is damaged and loses its command over the transportation of water dampness. These evil fluids accumulate and congeal into phlegm.

Main symptoms: Chest and lateral costal propping fullness, vertigo, heart palpitations, possible shortness of breath and coughing, possible progressive emaciation

Tongue & coating: A white, slimy tongue coating

Pulse image: A wiry, slippery or deep, tight pulse

Treatment principles: Warm and transform phlegm rheum, fortify the spleen and disinhibit dampness

Rx: *Ling Gui Zhu Gan Tang* (Poria, Cinnamon, Atractylodes & Licorice Decoction)

Ingredients:

Sclerotium Poriae Cocos (*Fu Ling*)
Ramulus Cinnamomi (*Gui Zhi*)

Rhizoma Atractylodis Macrocephalae (*Bai Zhu*)
Radix Glycyrrhizae (*Gan Cao*)

Additions & subtractions: For excessive phlegm, add Fructus Perillae Frutescentis (*Su Zi*), Semen Lepedii (*Ting Li Zi*), and Fructus Zizyphi Jujubae (*Da Zao*). For vomiting watery fluids and phlegm, add Rhizoma Pinelliae Ternatae (*Ban Xia*) and Pericarpium Citri Reticulatae (*Chen Pi*). For glomus and pain in the epigastrium, add Fructus Aurantii (*Zhi Ke*) and Cortex Magnoliae Officinalis (*Hou Po*).

Acupuncture & moxibustion: *Pi Shu* (Sp 20), *Zhong Wan* (CV 12), *Gong Sun* (Sp 4), *Nei Guan* (Per 6), *Zu San Li* (St 36), *Yin Ling Quan* (Sp 9)

Key advice: this pattern is also called phlegm rheum in the stomach and intestines.

If the kidney qi is weak and unable to steam and transform fluids, in order to warm the kidneys and disinhibit water, use *Ji Sheng Shen Qi Wan* (*Aid the Living* Kidney Qi Pills): prepared Radix Rehmanniae (*Shu Di*), Radix Dioscoreae Oppositae (*Shan Yao*), Fructus Corni Officinalis (*Shan Zhu Yu*), Cortex Radicis Moutan (*Dan Pi*), Sclerotium Poriae Cocos (*Fu Ling*), Rhizoma Alismatis (*Ze Xie*), Radix Lateralis Praeparatus Aconiti Carmichaeli (*Fu Zi*), Cortex Cinnamomi (*Rou Gui*), Semen Plantaginis (*Che Qian Zi*), Radix Cyathulae (*Chuan Niu Xi*).

If evil water is more prominent than visceral vacuity and there is a hidden pulse, an urge to move the bowels after which the patient feels better but a continuing fullness and distention in the upper abdomen, this is called lingering rheum and should be treated with *Gan Sui Ban Xia Tang* (Euphorbia & Pinellia Decoction): Radix Euphorbiae Kansui (*Gan Sui*), Rhizoma Pinelliae Ternatae (*Ban Xia*), Radix Albus Paeoniae Lactiflorae (*Bai Shao*), mix-fried Radix Glycyrrhizae (*Zhi Gan Cao*).

If rheum obstructs the intestines causing constipation, use *Ji Jiao Li Huang Wan* (Stephania, Zanthoxylum Croton & Rhubarb Pills): Radix Stephaniae Tetrandrae (*Han Fang Ji*), Fructus Zanthoxyli Bungeani (*Chuan Jiao*), Semen Crotonis Tiglii (*Ting Li Zi*), Radix Et Rhizoma Rhei (*Da Huang*).

If constipation is accompanied by abdominal fullness, use *Hou Po Da Huang Tang* (Magnolia & Rhubarb Decoction): Cortex Magnoliae Officinalis (*Hou Po*), Radix Et Rhizoma Rhei (*Da Huang*), Fructus Immaturus Aurantii (*Zhi Shi*).

Phlegm Evils

Phlegm Dampness

Disease causes, disease mechanisms: This pattern is due to overeating raw, chilled foods and sweet, fatty, thick-flavored foods possibly compounded by lack of exercise and excessive thinking or overtaxation. This may damage the spleen. the spleen thus loses fortification and its control over transportation and transformation. Hence dampness accumulates and congeals into phlegm.

Main symptoms: Excessive phlegm that is white in color and easily expectorated, chest and diaphragmatic glomus and oppression, nausea and vomiting, fatigue of the body and limbs, possible vertigo and palpitations

Tongue & coating: A white, moist, slimy tongue coating

Pulse image: A slippery pulse

Treatment principles: Dry dampness and transform phlegm, rectify the qi and harmonize the center

Rx: *Er Chen Tang* (Two Aged [Ingredients] Decoction)

Ingredients:

Rhizoma Pinelliae Ternatae (*Ban Xia*)
Pericarpium Citri Reticulatae (*Ju Pi*)
Sclerotium Poriae Cocos (*Bai Fu Ling*)
Radix Glycyrrhizae (*Gan Cao*)
uncooked Rhizoma Zingiberis (*Sheng Jiang*)
Fructus Pruni Mume (*Wu Mei*)

Additions & subtractions: For cold phlegm, add dry Rhizoma Zingiberis (*Gan Jiang*) and Herba Cum Radice Asari Sieboldi (*Xi Xin*). For hot phlegm, add Radix Scutellariae Baicalensis (*Huang Qin*), Semen Trichosanthis Kirlowii (*Gua Lou*), and Concretio Silicea Bambusae (*Tian Zhu Huang*). For wind phlegm, add bile(-treated) Rhizoma Arisaematis (*Dan Xing*) and Rhizoma Typhonii Gigantaeae (*Bai Fu Zi*). For phlegm complicated by food stagnation, add Semen Raphani Sativi (*Lai Fu Zi*).

Acupuncture & moxibustion: *Feng Long* (St 40), *Zu San Li* (St 36), *Zhong Wan* (CV 12), *Pi Shu* (Bl 20)

Key advice: This is a very general pattern. For more specific patterns relating to the accumulation of phlegm in various viscera, see Viscera & Bowel Pattern Discrimination above. For more specific patterns of phlegm accumulating in other parts of the body, see the patterns below.

Phlegm Lodged in the Chest & Lateral Costal Regions

Disease causes, disease mechanisms: This may be due to a combination of unregulated diet with too many raw, chilled foods and sweet, fatty, thick-flavored foods and anger and frustration causing qi stagnation. Because phlegm turbidity obstructs the free flow of yang qi in the chest, there is chest oppression and eventually chest pain. Because the qi mechanism is blocked and obstructed, there is shortness of breath, dyspnea, and rapid breathing. Because the spleen governs the four limbs and phlegm turbidity is affecting the spleen with consequent loss in the spleen's transportation, there is heaviness in the body and limbs and a fat body.

Main symptoms: Chest oppression eventually results in pain and this pain may stretch from the chest to the upper back or lateral coastal regions. This is accompanied by shortness of breath, dyspnea, and rapid breathing, heaviness in the body and limbs, a fat body, and excessive phlegm

Tongue & coating: A turbid, slimy tongue coating

Pulse image: Slippery

Treatment principles: Open yang and drain turbidity, wash away phlegm and open binding

Rx: *Gua Lou Xie Bai Ban Xia Tang Jia Wei* (Trichosanthes, Allium & Pinellia Decoction with Added Flavors)

Ingredients:

Fructus Trichosanthis Kirlowii (*Gua Lou*)
Bulbus Allii (*Xie Bai*)

Rhizoma Pinelliae Ternatae (*Ban Xia*)
dry Rhizoma Zingiberis (*Gan Jiang*)
Pericarpium Citri Reticulatae (*Chen Pi*)
Fructus Cardamomi (*Bai Kou Ren*)
White, *i.e.*, Grain, Alcohol (*Bai Jiu*)

Acupuncture & moxibustion: *Shan Zhong* (CV 17), *Zhong Wan* (CV 12), *Da Bao* (Sp 21), *Nei Guan* (Per 6), *Feng Long* (St 40), *Shen Dao* (GV 11)

Key advice: This pattern is similar to phlegm blocking the heart. Patients presenting with chest pain should always be referred to a Western physician for diagnosis and monitoring just to be safe.

Phlegm & Qi Joining & Obstructing

Disease causes, disease mechanisms: This pattern is mostly due to anger, stress, and frustration causing liver depression, qi stagnation. The qi stagnates and accumulates and then counterflows upward. In this case, there is also excessive phlegm due to weak spleen function. The spleen may be damaged by overeating raw, chilled foods or sweet, fatty, thick-flavored foods. It may also be damaged by too little exercise, overthinking and worry, or overtaxation. Because of the spleen's loss of control over transportation and transformation, dampness accumulates and, if it endures, it congeals into phlegm. When the qi counterflows upward, it drafts along with it this phlegm, which then lodges in the throat.

Main symptoms: The patient feels a foreign body like a plum pit or piece of meat obstructing their throat. This is can neither be spit out nor swallowed down. The patient will usually agree that they are excessively phlegmy.

Tongue & coating: A white, slimy tongue coating

Pulse image: A wiry, slippery, wiry, fine, or soggy pulse

Treatment principles: Course the liver and fortify the spleen, downbear counterflow and transform phlegm

Rx: *Si Qi Tang* (Four [Ingredients for the] Seven [Affects] Decoction)

Ingredients:

Rhizoma Pinelliae Ternatae (*Ban Xia*)
Cortex Magnoliae Officinalis (*Hou Po*)
Sclerotium Poriae Cocos (*Fu Ling*)
uncooked Rhizoma Zingiberis (*Sheng Jiang*)
Folium Perillae Frutescentis (*Su Ye*)
Fructus Zizyphi Jujubae (*Da Zao*)

Additions & subtractions: If there is chest distention and oppression and sighing, add Radix Bupleuri (*Chai Hu*), Radix Albus Paeoniae Lactiflorae (*Bai Shao*), and Rhizoma Cyperi Rotundi (*Xiang Fu*). For wandering pain of the body, add Fructus Meliae Toosendan (*Chuan Lian Zi*) and Tuber Curcumae (*Yu Jin*).

Acupuncture & moxibustion: *Nei Guan* (Per 6), *Gong Sun* (Sp 4), *Zhong Wan* (CV 12), *Shan Zhong* (CV 17), *Tian Tu* (CV 22), *Feng Long* (St 40)

Key advice: This pattern is also called plum pit qi. Western patients may not respond to the Chinese descriptions of a foreign object stuck in the throat. They usually describe the sensation as post-nasal drip. Western medicine classifies this condition as neurotic esophageal stenosis. This underscores this conditions association with stress and frustration damaging the liver. When there is plum pit qi, there is always a combination of phlegm and upwardly counterflow qi. This pattern only describes the combination of liver depression with phlegm accumulation obstructing the throat. There may also be more complex patterns associated with yin vacuity and blood stasis.

Phlegm Pit Scrofula

Disease causes, disease mechanisms: Phlegm pit scrofula is usually due to the same sorts of causes and mechanisms a work in plum pit qi. However, instead of lodging within the throat, it lodges in the flesh and muscle under the jaws and around the neck.

Main symptoms: Swollen lymph nodes in the neck

Tongue & coating: A thin, white, slimy tongue coating

Pulse image: A slippery, wiry pulse

Treatment principles: Transform phlegm and soften the hard, scatter nodulation and open the network vessels

Rx: *Xia Ku Cao Gao* (Prunella Syrup)

Ingredients:

Spica Prunellae Vulgaris (*Xia Ku Cao*)
Radix Angelicae Sinensis (*Dang Gui*)
Radix Albus Paeoniae Lactiflorae (*Bai Shao*)
Radix Scrophulariae Ningpoensis (*Xuan Shen*)
Radix Linderae Strychnifoliae (*Wu Yao*)
Bulbus Fritillariae Thunbergii (*Zhe Bei Mu*)
Bombyx Batryticatus (*Jiang Can*)
Thallus Algae (*Kun Bu*)
Radix Platycodi Grandiflori (*Jie Geng*)
Pericarpium Citri Reticulatae (*Chen Pi*)
Radix Ligustici Wallichii (*Chuan Xiong*)
Radix Glycyrrhizae (*Gan Cao*)
Rhizoma Cyperi Rotundi (*Xiang Fu*)
Flos Carthami Tinctorii (*Hong Hua*)
Fructus Zizyphi Jujubae (*Da Zao*)

Additions & subtractions: For increased efficacy in softening the hard, add Concha Ostreae (*Mu Li*) and Herba Sargassii (*Hai Zao*). If there is marked spleen vacuity, add Radix Astragali Membranacei (*Huang Qi*) and Radix Codonopsis Pilosulae (*Dang Shen*).

Acupuncture & moxibustion: *Shao Hai* (Ht 3), *Tian Jing* (TB 10), *Feng Long* (St 40), *Pi Shu* (Sp 20), *Bai Lao* (M-HN-30)

Key advice: This pattern covers lymphadenopathy, goiter, and nodules on the thyroid.

Phlegm Nodulation with Qi & Blood Dual Vacuity

Disease causes, disease mechanisms: It is qi that transforms and engenders the blood and that moves and transports the blood and body fluids. Therefore, qi vacuity due to enduring disease may lead to blood vacuity and also to blood stasis. Because the qi is vacuous and weak, it may fail to transport and transform fluids and humors. This is all the more likely when, due to blood vacuity, the qi fails to flow smoothly and uninhibitedly. Therefore, fluids and humors may accumulate and congeal into phlegm. Because the blood and body fluids flow together throughout the body, if the blood becomes static it may impede the flow of body fluids and also contribute to their turning into phlegm nodulations.

Main symptoms: Swellings and kernels in the neck, lack of strength of the four limbs, a pale, white facial complexion, dizziness, blurred vision, emaciation, fatigued spirit, scanty appetite, shortness of breath on moving

Tongue & coating: A thin, slimy tongue coating

Pulse image: A fine, forceless, possibly soggy pulse

Treatment principles: Greatly supplement the qi and blood, transform phlegm and scatter nodulation

Rx: *Xiang Bei Yang Ying Wan Jia Jian* (Fritillaria Nourish the Constructive Pills with Additions & Subtractions)

Ingredients:

prepared Radix Rehmanniae (*Shu Di*)
Radix Angelicae Sinensis (*Dang Gui*)
Radix Albus Paeoniae Lactiflorae (*Bai Shao*)
Radix Ligustici Wallichii (*Chuan Xiong*)
Radix Panacis Ginseng (*Ren Shen*)
Rhizoma Atractylodis Macrocephalae (*Bai Zhu*)
Sclerotium Poriae Cocos (*Fu Ling*)
mix-fried Radix Glycyrrhizae (*Zhi Gan Cao*)
Rhizoma Cyperi Rotundi (*Xiang Fu*)
Bulbus Fritillariae Thunbergii (*Zhe Bei Mu*)
Rhizoma Dioscoreae Bulbiferae (*Huang Yao Zi*)
Radix Semiaquilegiae (*Tian Kui Zi*)
calcined Concha Ostreae (*Mu Li*)
Pericarpium Citri Reticulatae (*Chen Pi*)
uncooked Rhizoma Zingiberis (*Sheng Jiang*)
Fructus Zizyphi Jujubae (*Da Zao*)

Acupuncture & moxibustion: *Tian Jing* (TB 10), *Bai Lao* (M-HN-30), *Zu San Li* (St 36), *San Yin Jiao* (Sp 6), *Da Zhui* (GV 14), *Ge Shu* (Bl 17), *Pi Shu* (Bl 20), *Shen Shu* (Bl 23)

Phlegm Nodulation with Yin Vacuity, Internal Heat

Disease causes, disease mechanisms: If there is yin vacuity due to enduring disease, this may give rise internal heat. Whereas enduring internal heat may give rise to yin vacuity. In either case, such vacuous heat may counterflow upward, stewing the juices and congealing those into phlegm. This phlegm may then be drafted along with this upward counterflow to lodge in the neck, the back of the head, or under the arms, forming phlegm nodulations.

Main symptoms: Generalized swollen lymph glands, tidal fever, night sweats, vacuity vexation, loss of sleep, dizziness and tinnitus, lassitude of the spirit, vexatious heat in the five hearts, a dry mouth

Tongue & coating: A red tongue with a scanty, yellowish coating

Pulse image: Fine and rapid

Treatment principles: Enrich yin and downbear fire, soften the hard and scatter nodulation

Rx: *Da Bu Yin Wan Jia Jian* (Great Supplement Yin Pills with Additions & Subtractions)

Ingredients:

Rhizoma Anemarrhenae (*Zhi Mu*)
Cortex Phellodendri (*Huang Bai*)
prepared Radix Rehmanniae (*Shu Di*)
Plastrum Testudinis (*Gui Ban*)
Radix Scrophulariae Ningpoensis (*Xuan Shen*)
Bulbus Fritillariae Thunbergii (*Zhe Bei Mu*)
Spica Prunellae Vulgaris (*Xia Ku Cao*)
Herba Sargassii (*Hai Zao*)
Thallus Algae (*Kun Bu*)
Radix Glycyrrhizae (*Gan Cao*)

Acupuncture & moxibustion: *Tian Jing* (TB 10), *Shao Hai* (Ht 3), *Bai Lao* (M-HN-30), *Shen Shu* (Bl 23), *Tai Xi* (Ki 3), *San Yin Jiao* (Sp 6)

Key advice: Here there are swollen lymph nodes but accompanied by more prominent signs and symptoms of yin vacuity and internal heat.

Phlegm & Stasis Mutually Obstructing

Disease causes, disease mechanisms: Blood and body fluids share a common source and flow together throughout the body. Enduring phlegm obstruction may eventually cause blood stasis, while enduring blood stasis may eventually result in phlegm accumulation and nodulation.

Main symptoms: Swollen lymph nodes all over the body or other nodulations that are firm and immovable when pressed

Tongue & coating: A dark, purple tongue

Pulse image: A wiry, choppy pulse

Treatment principles: Transform phlegm and soften the hard, dispel stasis and open the network vessels

Rx: *Xi Huang Wan Jia Jian* (Synthetic Bezoar Pills with Additions & Subtractions)

Ingredients:

Resina Olibani (*Ru Xiang*)
Resina Myrrhae (*Mo Yao*)
Calculus Bovis Syntheticus (*Xi Huang*)
Secretio Moschi Moschiferi (*She Xiang*)
Radix Scrophulariae Ningpoensis (*Xuan Shen*)
Spica Prunellae Vulgaris (*Xia Ku Cao*)
Bulbus Fritillariae Thunbergii (*Zhe Bei Mu*)
Radix Ranunculi Ternatae (*Mao Gua Cao*)
Rhizoma Dioscoreae Bulbiferae (*Huang Yao Zi*)
ginger[-processed] Rhizoma Pinelliae Ternatae (*Ban Xia*)
uncooked Concha Ostreae (*Mu Li*)

Radix Paridis Polyphyllae (*Zai Xiu*)
processed Rhizoma Arisaematis (*Nan Xing*)

Acupuncture & moxibustion: *Tian Jing* (TB 10), *Qu Chi* (LI 11), *Feng Long* (ST 40), *Xue Hai* (Sp 10), *Ge Shu* (Bl 17)

Key advice: This pattern may be observed in cases of thyroid tumors, Kaposi's sarcoma, and various uterine and ovarian tumors.

Phlegm and stasis may also obstruct the channels and network vessels. In that case, there may be symptoms as mild as numbness or as severe as paralysis. This is often due to enduring wind, damp, cold *bi*. In this case, the tongue is purplish or has static spots or macules and it has a slimy coating. For patients with a strong bodily constitution, use *Da Huo Luo Dan* (Great Quickening the Network Vessels Elixir [available as a ready-made patent medicine]). For patients who are concomitantly vacuous and weak, use *Xiao Huo Luo Dan* (Minor Quickening the Network Vessels Elixir): processed Radix Aconiti (*Chuan Wu*), processed Radix Aconiti Kusnezoffi (*Cao Wu*), bile-processed Rhizoma Arisaematis (*Dan Nan Xing*), Resina Olibani (*Ru Xiang*), Resina Myrrhae (*Mo Yao*), and Lumbricus (*Di Long*).

Phlegm Turbidity Obstructing the Middle

Disease causes, disease mechanisms: This pattern is due to spleen vacuity losing control over the transportation and transformation of body fluids. Such spleen vacuity with accumulation of dampness may be due to overeating raw, chilled and sweet, fatty, thick-flavored foods typically combined with lack of adequate exercise, overtaxation, and excessive thinking. Dampness and phlegm accumulate and obstruct the free and uninhibited flow of qi. Thus qi accumulates and eventually counterflows upward as wind. This wind drafts with it phlegm and dampness or turbidity, which block the clear portals, producing headache and dizziness.

Main symptoms: Dizziness, vertigo, headache like a tight band squeezing the head, chest oppression, vomiting, nausea, excessive phlegm

Tongue & coating: A white, slimy tongue coating

Pulse image: A wiry, slippery or soft, slippery pulse

Treatment principles: Dry dampness and transform phlegm, level the liver and extinguish wind

Rx: *Ban Xia Bai Zhu Tian Ma Tang* (Pinellia, Atractylodes & Gastrodia Decoction)

Ingredients:

Rhizoma Pinelliae Ternatae (*Ban Xia*)
Rhizoma Gastrodiae Elatae (*Tian Ma*)
Sclerotium Poriae Cocos (*Fu Ling*)
Exocarpium Citri Rubri (*Ju Hong*)
Rhizoma Atractylodis Macrocephalae (*Bai Zhu*)
Radix Glycyrrhizae (*Gan Cao*)
uncooked Rhizoma Zingiberis (*Sheng Jiang*)
Fructus Zizyphi Jujubae (*Da Zao*)

Additions & subtractions: For severe dizziness and vertigo, add Bombyx Batryticatus (*Jiang Can*) and bile(-treated) Rhizoma Arisaematis (*Dan Nan Xing*). For frontal headache, add Radix Angelicae Dahuricae (*Bai Zhi*). For severe headache, add Fructus Viticis (*Man Jing Zi*). For symptoms of hot phlegm, add Caulis Bambusae In Taeniis (*Zhu Ru*).

Acupuncture & moxibustion: *Nei Guan* (Per 6), *Bai Hui* (GV 20), *Feng Long* (St 40), *Zhong Wan* (CV 12), *Yin Ling Quan* (Sp 9)

Key advice: This headache is frequently accompanied by nausea. However, any severely painful headache may be accompanied by nausea. Here, the pain is like a tight band squeezing around the head and the head feels full, heavy, and clouded. In addition, there are usually prominent symptoms of spleen dampness and even spleen vacuity, such as reduced appetite, loose stools, and fatigue. Further, the patient typically reports excessive phlegm and possibly even plum pit qi.

the more likely when, due to blood vacuity, the qi fails to flow smoothly and uninhibitedly. Therefore, fluids and humors may accumulate and congeal into phlegm. Because the blood and body fluids flow together throughout the body, if the blood becomes static it may impede the flow of body fluids and also contribute to their turning into phlegm nodulations.

Main symptoms: Swellings and kernels in the neck, lack of strength of the four limbs, a pale, white facial complexion, dizziness, blurred vision, emaciation, fatigued spirit, scanty appetite, shortness of breath on moving

Tongue & coating: A thin, slimy tongue coating

Pulse image: A fine, forceless, possibly soggy pulse

Treatment principles: Greatly supplement the qi and blood, transform phlegm and scatter nodulation

Rx: *Xiang Bei Yang Ying Wan Jia Jian* (Fritillaria Nourish the Constructive Pills with Additions & Subtractions)

Ingredients:

prepared Radix Rehmanniae (*Shu Di*)
Radix Angelicae Sinensis (*Dang Gui*)
Radix Albus Paeoniae Lactiflorae (*Bai Shao*)
Radix Ligustici Wallichii (*Chuan Xiong*)
Radix Panacis Ginseng (*Ren Shen*)
Rhizoma Atractylodis Macrocephalae (*Bai Zhu*)
Sclerotium Poriae Cocos (*Fu Ling*)
mix-fried Radix Glycyrrhizae (*Zhi Gan Cao*)
Rhizoma Cyperi Rotundi (*Xiang Fu*)
Bulbus Fritillariae Thunbergii (*Zhe Bei Mu*)
Rhizoma Dioscoreae Bulbiferae (*Huang Yao Zi*)
Radix Semiaquilegiae (*Tian Kui Zi*)
calcined Concha Ostreae (*Mu Li*)
Pericarpium Citri Reticulatae (*Chen Pi*)
uncooked Rhizoma Zingiberis (*Sheng Jiang*)
Fructus Zizyphi Jujubae (*Da Zao*)

Treatment principles: Transform phlegm and soften the hard, scatter nodulation and open the network vessels

Rx: *Xia Ku Cao Gao* (Prunella Syrup)

Ingredients:

Spica Prunellae Vulgaris (*Xia Ku Cao*)
Radix Angelicae Sinensis (*Dang Gui*)
Radix Albus Paeoniae Lactiflorae (*Bai Shao*)
Radix Scrophulariae Ningpoensis (*Xuan Shen*)
Radix Linderae Strychnifoliae (*Wu Yao*)
Bulbus Fritillariae Thunbergii (*Zhe Bei Mu*)
Bombyx Batryticatus (*Jiang Can*)
Thallus Algae (*Kun Bu*)
Radix Platycodi Grandiflori (*Jie Geng*)
Pericarpium Citri Reticulatae (*Chen Pi*)
Radix Ligustici Wallichii (*Chuan Xiong*)
Radix Glycyrrhizae (*Gan Cao*)
Rhizoma Cyperi Rotundi (*Xiang Fu*)
Flos Carthami Tinctorii (*Hong Hua*)
Fructus Zizyphi Jujubae (*Da Zao*)

Additions & subtractions: For increased efficacy in softening the hard, add Concha Ostreae (*Mu Li*) and Herba Sargassii (*Hai Zao*). If there is marked spleen vacuity, add Radix Astragali Membranacei (*Huang Qi*) and Radix Codonopsis Pilosulae (*Dang Shen*).

Acupuncture & moxibustion: *Shao Hai* (Ht 3), *Tian Jing* (TB 10), *Feng Long* (St 40), *Pi Shu* (Sp 20), *Bai Lao* (M-HN-30)

Key advice: This pattern covers lymphadenopathy, goiter, and nodules on the thyroid.

Phlegm Nodulation with Qi & Blood Dual Vacuity

Disease causes, disease mechanisms: It is qi that transforms and engenders the blood and that moves and transports the blood and body fluids. Therefore, qi vacuity due to enduring disease may lead to blood vacuity and also to blood stasis. Because the qi is vacuous and weak, it may fail to transport and transform fluids and humors. This is all

5
Channel & Network Vessel Pattern Discrimination

Under this heading, we only present those patterns associated with *bi zheng* or blockage condition. In the previous chapters we have discussed cold in the liver channel, depressive heat in the heart channel, phlegm and stasis mutually binding and obstructing the channels and network vessels, an so on. Although acupuncture texts give the signs and symptoms of repletion and vacuity of each of the 12 regular channels, they do not typically give specific treatment protocols for each of these. Neither do Chinese internal medicine texts discuss these; therefore, we have not included them here.

Wind Striking the Channels & Network Vessels

Disease causes, disease mechanisms: If wind evils enter the channels, they may block and obstruct the free and smooth flow of qi and blood, thus giving rise to symptoms of aching and pain, limited motion, and possible spasm or numbness.

Main symptoms: Migratory joint pain, especially of the wrists, elbows, knees, and ankles, possible deviation of the eye and mouth, hemiplegia

Tongue & coating: A thin, white tongue coating, *i.e.*, no particular abnormal tongue changes

Pulse image: A floating pulse

Treatment principles: Dispel wind and open the channels

Rx: *Fang Feng Tang Jia Jian* (Ledebouriella Decoction with Additions & Subtractions)

Ingredients:

Radix Ledebouriellae Sesloidis (*Fang Feng*)
Radix Angelicae Sinensis (*Dang Gui*)

Radix Gentianae Macrophyllae (*Qin Jiao*)
Radix Puerariae (*Ge Gen*)
Radix Ephedrae (*Ma Huang*)
Radix Et Rhizoma Notopterygii (*Qiang Huo*)
Herba Seu Flos Schizonepetae Tenuifoliae (*Jing Jie Sui*)
Caulis Milletiae Seu Spatholobi (*Ji Xue Tang*)
Caulis Trachelospermi (*Luo Shi Teng*)

Acupuncture & moxibustion: *Feng Fu* (GV 16), *Feng Men* (Bl 12), *Da Zhui* (GV 14), *Feng Chi* (GB 20), *Tai Chong* (Liv 3), *He Gu* (LI 4), and *Qu Chi* (LI 11) plus local points on the affected channels and *a shi* points

Key advice: External wind evils almost always combine with other of the six environmental excesses. Thus the treatment principles given above include eliminating dampness. Wind dampness is the Chinese name for rheumatic complaints. When encountered by itself, this pattern may also be called moving *bi*.

Dampness Striking the Channels & Network Vessels

Disease causes, disease mechanisms: If one lies on damp ground, works immersed in water, or is caught in the rain, dampness may invade the body, lodging in the channels and network vessels and causing damp *bi*, swelling, and pain.

Main symptoms: Numbness, fixed joint pain aggravated by exposure to dampness and low pressure weather systems, possible swelling of the affected area

Tongue & coating: A slimy, white tongue coating

Pulse image: A slippery, slow pulse

Treatment principles: Eliminate dampness and open the channels

Rx: *Yi Yi Ren Tang Jia Jian* (Coix Decoction with Additions & Subtractions)

Ingredients:

Radix Ligustici Wallichii (*Chuan Xiong*)
Rhizoma Atractylodis (*Cang Zhu*)
Radix Et Rhizoma Notopterygii (*Qiang Huo*)

170

Albus Paeoniae Lactiflorae (*Bai Shao*)
Astragali Membranacei (*Huang Qi*)
Glycyrrhizae (*Gan Cao*)
ed Radix Lateralis Praeparatus Aconiti Carmichaeli (*Fu Zi*)
izoma Zingiberis (*Gan Jiang*)
Cum Radice Asari Sieboldi (*Xi Xin*)
us Cinnamomi (*Gui Zhi*)

incture & moxibustion: *Da Zhui* (GV 14), *Shen Que* (CV 8), *Ming Men* (GV 4), *Chi* (TB 4), and *Chong Yang* (St 42) plus points on the course of the affected ls and *a shi* points

dvice: Often wind, cold, and dampness invade together. However, sometimes one : simple cold *bi* pain. Cold constricts and congeals the flow of qi and blood, giving concomitant blood stasis.

Damp *Bi* of the Channels & Network Vessels

se causes, disease mechanisms: If wind and dampness invade the body, they dge in the channels and network vessels, thus obstructing the flow of qi and blood. en gives rise to pain, limited movement, and possible swelling.

symptoms: A heavy painful head, bodily heaviness, joint pain that comes and goes tuates in intensity but tends to strike the same location every time, pain worsened np weather

ue & coating: A white coating

image: A floating, possibly wiry pulse

nent principles: Dispel wind and eliminate dampness

iang Huo Sheng Shi Tang (Notopterygium Overcome Dampness Decoction)

dients:

Et Rhizoma Notopterygii (*Qiang Huo*)
Angelicae Pubescentis (*Du Huo*)
na Et Radix Ligustici Sinensis (*Gao Ben*)

Radix Angelicae Pubescentis (*Du Huo*)
Radix Ledebouriellae Sesloidis (*Fang Feng*)
Radix Aconiti (*Chuan Wu Tou*)
Herba Ephedrae (*Ma Huang*)
Ramulus Cinnamomi (*Gui Zhi*)
Radix Angelicae Sinensis (*Dang Gui*)
Radix Stephaniae Tetrandrae (*Fang Ji*)
Rhizoma Dioscoreae Hypoglaucae (*Bi Xie*)
Semen Coicis Lachryma-jobi (*Yi Yi Ren*)

Acupuncture & moxibustion: *Yin Ling Quan* (Sp 9), *San Yin Ji*
20), *Pang Guang Shu* (Bl 28), and *Shui Quan* (Ki 5) plus local point
affected channels and *a shi* points

Key advice: This pattern is not so commonly seen in clinical pract
or wind, cold, and dampness. When encountered, a clear, bland, sp
extremely important, as is avoiding chilled and raw foods. This patte
bi or fixed *bi*.

Cold Striking the Channels & Network Vessels

Disease causes, disease mechanisms: Cold evils may en
network vessels where they obstruct the flow of qi and blood, thus

Main symptoms: Severe, stabbing pain in the joints, fixed pain
obtains warmth and worsens on exposure to cold

Tongue & coating: A thin, white coating

Pulse image: A wiry or tight pulse

Treatment principles: Warm the channels and scatter cold

Rx: *Da Wu Tou Tang Jia Jian* (*Wu Tou* Aconite Decoction with Add

Ingredients:

Radix Aconiti (*Chuan Wu Tou*)
Herba Ephedrae (*Ma Huang*)

Radix Ledebouriellae Sesloidis (*Fang Feng*)
Radix Ligustici Wallichii (*Chuan Xio*ng)
Fructus Viticis (*Man Jing Zi*)
mix-fried Radix Glycyrrhizae (*Zhi Gan Cao*)

Additions & subtractions: If there is severe pain due to complication by cold, add Radix Lateralis Praeparatus Aconiti Carmichaeli (*Fu Zi*).

Acupuncture & moxibustion: *Wai Guan* (TB 5), *He Gu* (LI 4), *Yin Ling Quan* (Sp 9), *Zu San Li* (St 36), and *Zhi Yang* (GV 9) plus local points on the course of the affected channels and *a shi* points

Key advice: If wind damp *bi* endures, it will result in both blood stasis and possible phlegm obstruction. In addition, qi stagnation may transform into localized heat.

Damp Heat in the Channels & Network Vessels

Disease causes, disease mechanisms: Due to either external invasion by damp heat, depressive heat transforming dampness, or spleen vacuity transforming heat, damp heat may obstruct and block the channels and network vessels.

Main symptoms: Swelling, erythema, a hot sensation, and pain in the joints and skin primarily of the lower limbs accompanied by bodily heaviness, lassitude, fever, slight sweating, poor appetite, chest oppression, a sallow yellow facial complexion, loose stools

Tongue & coating: A red tongue with a slimy, yellow coating

Pulse image: A slippery, rapid pulse

Treatment principles: Clear heat and eliminate dampness

Rx: *Er Miao San Jia Jian* (Two Wonders Powder with Additions & Subtractions)

Ingredients:

Cortex Phellodendri (*Huang Bai*)
Rhizoma Atractylodis (*Cang Zhu*)
Rhizoma Atractylodis Macrocephalae (*Bai Zhu*)

Radix Clematidis Chinensis (*Wei Ling Xian*)
Rhizoma Smilacis Glabrae (*Tu Fu Ling*)
Semen Coicis Lachryma-jobi (*Yi Yi Ren*)
Radix Angelicae Pubescentis (*Du Huo*)
Radix Et Rhizoma Notopterygii (*Qiang Huo*)
Radix Sophorae Flavescentis (*Ku Shen*)
Cortex Radicis Acanthopanacis (*Wu Jia Pi*)

Acupuncture & moxibustion: *Yin Ling Quan* (Sp 9), *Qu Chi* (LI 11), *Yang Ling Quan* (GB 34), *Wai Guan* (TB 5) or *Zhi Gou* (TB 6) plus local points along the course of the affected channels and *a shi* points

Key advice: Whenever there is damp heat, what the Chinese call a clear, bland diet is very important. Sweets, fatty foods, thick-flavored foods, acrid, peppery, hot foods, and alcohol are all contraindicated.

If damp heat endures, it will do any of several things. It may block and obstruct the flow of qi and blood, thus causing stagnation and stasis. Heat may consume and damage yin fluids, giving rise to simultaneous yin vacuity, vacuity heat signs and symptoms. And it may damage the liver and kidneys, giving rise to liver blood and kidney yang vacuity.

Conclusion
Tips on Discriminating Complex Patterns

The problem of complex patterns in real-life patients

Books on TCM pattern discrimination such as this are designed to separate out a number of different patterns for maximum clarity and ease of differentiation, one pattern from the other. However, in actual clinical practice, patients, and especially Western patients suffering from what are usually called difficult to treat, knotty diseases, do not typically present with such neat, discreet patterns. In our experience, most patients present complex patterns made up from several different co-existing patterns. This makes TCM pattern discrimination in clinical practice more difficult than books such as this imply.

In this book, we have tried to give more than the usual simple patterns, including a number of complex, but nevertheless commonly encountered complicated patterns. However, no book can give a completely exhaustive account of all the ways patterns can combine and vary in real-life patients. Therefore, students are cautioned to keep in mind that often there are at least two simultaneous or concomitant patterns presenting in patients with either chronic diseases, or certainly in acute diseases superimposed on chronic disease patterns.

Taking TCM theory as one's guide

Happily, not every pattern can combine with every other pattern. There are certain disease mechanisms that tend to evolve in certain ways, making certain complex patterns appear but not others. For instance, because cold is a yin evil that causes constriction and congelation, wind, cold, damp *bi* may eventually become complicated by phlegm and blood stasis due to cold's effect on the yang qi, which moves the blood on the one hand and transports and transforms fluids on the other. Or, due to Liu Wan-su's theory of similar transformation (*tong hua*), wind, cold, damp *bi* causing depression may transform into heat *bi*.

Likewise, most adults suffer from some degree of liver depression, qi stagnation. This has to do with the stress of being an adult with all the responsibilities that entails—breadwinner, parent, participating member of a community, filial child of one's aging parents, and so on. However, based on Chinese medical theory, we know that the liver has certain relationships with other viscera and bowels. Therefore, it should be no hard conceptual leap to understand either liver/stomach disharmony, liver/spleen disharmony, liver/lung disharmony, liver/heart depressive heat, liver blood/kidney yin vacuity, liver blood/kidney yang vacuity, liver blood/kidney yin and yang vacuity, qi stagnation/blood stasis, qi stagnation/food retention, qi stagnation/ damp depression, qi stagnation/blood vacuity, etc.

Further, certain complications can be explained by an individual's sex. For instance, in women, the monthly menstruation is a loss of blood that makes the arising of liver qi even more probable, since it is blood that softens and harmonizes the liver. Since the spleen is the postnatal root of blood engenderment and transformation, it is no wonder that women are prone to liver depression/spleen vacuity. Since blood nourishes the heart and quiets the spirit, it should also be no wonder to see liver depression, spleen qi vacuity, and heart blood vacuity. Again, since the spleen is the middle source of water, it should come as no surprise that phlegm dampness might also complicate this scenario.

Other complications can be explained based on age. In women in their 20s and early 30s, it is most common to see liver depression, spleen vacuity, and blood vacuity. However, by the mid to late 30s and on through the 40s, most women suffer from elements of liver depression, blood vacuity, spleen qi vacuity, *and* kidney yang vacuity with possible heat in the stomach, heart, and/or lungs. In the elderly, there is usually kidney vacuity, but also blood stasis, perhaps in the network vessels, and there may also be phlegm mutually binding with this stasis and obstructing.

Pattern discriminations are only working hypotheses

When studying acupuncture at the Shanghai college of TCM in 1982–1983, I once asked one of my teachers how to do a pattern discrimination for a real-life, difficult, and complex case. She said to analyze each sign and symptom one by one, listing all the possible disease mechanisms that could account for each one. What happens if one does this is that one will see certain disease mechanisms that are common to more than one sign or symptom. These common mechanisms are the ones most likely to be at work in the patient.

Based on this preliminary assessment, one forms a hypothesis about the patient's pattern. Then one checks to see if the patient does actually have other of the expected signs and symptoms of the suspected pattern. If the tongue and pulse, signs and symptoms corroborate that hypothesis, then one should give treatment on that basis.

However, one should be clear that the initial diagnosis is nothing other than a working hypothesis. As one of my first Chinese medicine teachers, Dr. (Eric) Tao Xi-yu, was fond of saying, the initial diagnosis is only a supposition. It is the result of treatment that clarifies and validates or invalidates that initial hypothesis. If the patient gets better, one can assume the pattern discrimination was largely correct. If they do not respond or actually get worse, then it is clear the initial diagnosis was wrong.

Nevertheless, even if that happens, one is closer to the actual diagnosis, because now, through experimentation, one has proven at least one thing that the diagnosis is not. Therefore, one should not think that they must get the initial diagnosis correct every time. That is wonderful when it happens, but pattern discrimination is usually an evolving process of refinement based on hypothesis, experimentation (*i.e.*, treatment), outcome (*i.e.*, new facts), new hypothesis, refined treatment, outcome, new hypothesis, and so on.

Making use of the basics

Almost everything one needs to know to successfully discriminate patterns, we learn in the first year of acupuncture school. What I mean here is that, when analyzing signs and symptoms, we need to stick to the basics, those fundamental statements of fact that we all learn right at the beginning of our schooling in Chinese medicine.

For instance, we may or may not have had a course in TCM dermatology in our undergraduate education. But that really does not matter. When faced with a problem case or a disease with which we are not already familiar, *always the first thing to do is to analyze the signs and symptoms in terms of yin and yang and their subdivisions of hot and cold, exterior and interior, and vacuity and repletion.*

Recently, a new practitioner called me to ask about a case of vulvar intraepithelial neoplasia (VIN). She wanted to discuss the treatment of the case based on the presence of supposed deep-lying evils (*fu xie*). However, I kept coming back to questioning her about the way the vulvar lesion actually looked. What color was it? Was it moist or dry? Was it itchy, burning, painful, swollen, raised, hot or inflamed?

It turned out that the vulvar lesion was paler than the surrounding skin and was dry and rough. It was not wet or weeping, was not ulcerated, was not raised, and was not painful. It did itch. Sometimes the lesion was surrounded by skin that was redder than normal, but not all the time. I kept asking the practitioner to analyze those signs and symptoms using basic TCM facts. She kept telling me theory about viral diseases. Finally, we walked together through an analysis of the lesion itself, point by point.

The fact that it was paler than the surrounding skin suggests a yin condition as opposed to a yang condition. This is corroborated by the lack of pain and heat. In particular, it suggests local blood vacuity, since the red color of the skin is due to the presence of blood. Since it was dry and rough, this corroborates that there is insufficient blood to nourish the local skin. Now the question is, why is there a local blood vacuity?

It turned out that the patient's other generalized signs and symptoms added up to liver depression, qi stagnation with some blood stasis. This was evidenced by premenstrual irritability, breast distention and pain, and painful periods, which were worse if she drank coffee or beer, or when she was under stress. In addition, she had a wiry pulse and there were some blood clots.

Based on this information, we can make a pretty good hypothesis about this woman's TCM pattern and the disease mechanisms at work causing her vulvar intra epithelial neoplasia. Liver depression and qi stagnation easily give rise to blood stasis over time, since it is the qi that moves the blood and if the qi stops, the blood will stop. If there is liver depression, typically the liver invades the spleen causing an element of blood vacuity. Thus it is easy to understand how there could be blood vacuity failing to nourish the skin of the vulva. In fact, the patient did suffer from persistent fatigue, a qi vacuity symptom.

But what about the blood stasis? In TCM, itching may be due to wind or to blood stasis. Itching may be due to heat causing the qi to be out-thrust to move recklessly in the exterior, or it may be due to blood vacuity not nourishing and rooting the qi. Thus the qi counterflows upward and outward. Itching may also be due to static blood in the network vessels because it may be seen as a type of pain. Thus, it is my hypothesis that the red area around the dry, itchy, pale lesion was in fact static blood that had entered the network vessels. In this case, there is a somewhat systemic blood vacuity complicated by a local blood stasis, making the local blood vacuity all the worse.

If the working hypothesis is that the patient's pattern is one of liver depression/spleen vacuity with blood vacuity and static blood having entered the network vessels, then the TCM treatment principles are to course the liver and resolve depression, fortify the spleen and nourish the blood, quicken the blood and open the network vessels. Having stated those principles, it is easy to then choose a guiding formula for internal administration and modify it with additions and subtractions. It is also easy to decide upon a local, external application. We would want something that both nourishes the blood and moistens the skin as well as quickens the blood and opens the network vessels.

All of the above analyses and conclusions are based on information learned (or should be learned), if not in the first six months, at least in the first year of acupuncture/TCM school. One merely has to put that information into use in analyzing a patient's signs and symptoms in order to arrive at a pretty fair deduction about their patient's pattern. However, the keys are 1) to keep the basics firmly in mind and then 2) apply them in a systematic way, step by step. Just as the longest, most abstruse and obscure English word in the world is made up of nothing more than the 26 letters of the alphabet, the most complex pattern is made up of nothing other than the basic statements of fact of TCM.

As it turns out, liver depression and qi and blood vacuity are both known TCM patterns identified in the Chinese TCM literature with VIN, the other patterns being damp heat pouring downward and yin and yang loss of regulation. However, even without knowing this in advance, we could hit on the right treatment just by TCM pattern discrimination.

At the moment, this pattern discrimination is only a hypothesis since this patient has not yet been treated based on the principles in turn based on this pattern. However, it nonetheless exemplifies several things: 1) TCM patterns tend to exist in combinations, 2) TCM patterns tend to be more complicated than the textbooks suggest (for instance, the above case being complicated by blood stasis in the network vessels), and 3) TCM patterns, even when complex, are made up of simple building blocks analyzed and known by basic TCM theory.

Conclusion

As in most arts, mastery is based on gaining a thorough understanding of the basics·and then applying those basics in a rigorously consistent and step by step way. Eventually, after one has gained a lot of clinical experience, it may seem that one knows their patients' patterns all at one intuitive leap. However, real masters can usually explain exactly the process they used to arrive at their deductions, except that, in the case of a master, they arrive at that deduction very, very fast.

But whether fast or slow, it should always be remembered that it is TCM pattern discrimination, and treatment based on that patttern discrimination, which is safe and holistic, empowering and enlightening Chinese medicine. Thus, we believe, it is worth the effort to perfect this methodology in clinical practice.

Bibliography

Chinese language

"A Short Treatise on Liver Qi Vacuity Pattern," Chen Jia-xu & Yang Wei-yi, *Zhong Yi Za Zhi (Journal of Chinese Medicine)*, Vol. 35, #5, 1994, pp. 264-267

"Clinical Characteristics of Liver Qi Vacuity," Chen Jia-xu & Yang Wei-yi, *Bei Jing Zhong Yi (Beijing Chinese Medicine)*, Vol. 16, #5, 1993, p. 13

Jian Ming Zhong Yi Da Ci Dian (A Simple, Clear Chinese Medicine Dictionary), Chinese National Chinese Medicine Research Institute & Guang Zhou College of TCM, People's Health & Hygiene Press, Beijing, 1986

Lin Chuang Bian Zheng Shi Zhi Xue (A Study of Carrying Out Treatment on the Basis of the Clinical Discrimination of Patterns), Liu Bin, Science, Technology & Literature Press, Beijing, 1992

Shi Yong Zhong Yi Nei Ke Xue (A Study of Practical Chinese Medicine Internal Medicine), Huang Wen-dong, Shanghai Science & Technology Press, Shanghai, 1986

Shi Yong Zhong Yi Zhen Duan Xue (A Study of Practical Chinese Medicine Diagnosis), Liu Tie-tiao, Shanghai Science & Technology Press, Shanghai, 1988

"What is Meant by Lung Yang Vacuity," Wang De-chun, *Shan Xi Zhong Yi (Shanxi Chinese Medicine)*, Vol. 7, #10, 1986, pp. 433-434

Zhong Yi Bing Yin Bing Ji Xue (A Study of Disease Causes & Disease Mechanisms in Chinese Medicine), Song Lu-bing, Peoples Health & Hygiene Press, Beijing, 1987

Zhong Yi Nei Ke Xue (A Study of Chinese Medicine Internal Medicine), Zhanhg Bo-yu *et al.*, People's Health & Hygiene Press, Beijing, 1991

Zhong Yi Nei Ke Xue Jiang Yi (Teaching Materials for the Study of Chinese Medicine Internal Medicine), Shanghai College of TCM, Medicine & Medicinals Bureau Press, Hong Kong, 1982

Zhong Yi Nei Ke Zheng Zhuang Bian Zhi Shou Ce (A Handbook of Chinese Medicine Internal Medicine Symptoms, Discrimination & Treatment), Fang Wen-xian, Liu Qing & Chu Xiu-jun, China Standard Press, Beijing, 1989

Zhong Yi Zheng Hou Zhen Duan Zhi Liao Xue (A Study of Chinese Medicine Patterns, Diagnosis & Treatment), Cheng Shao-en & Xia Hong-sheng, Beijing Science & Technology Press, Beijing, 1993

Zhong Yi Zheng Zhuang Jian Bie Zhen Duan Xue (A Study of Chinese Medicine Discrimination & Diagnosis), Zhao Jin-ze, People's Health & Hygiene Press, Beijing, 1984

Zhong Yi Zhi Liao Xue (A Study of Treatment in Chinese Medicine), Sun Guo-jie & Tu Jin-wen, Chinese Medicine Science & Technology Press, Beijing, 1990

English language

A Comprehensive Guide to Chinese Herbal Medicine, Ze-lin Chen & Mei-fang Chen, Oriental Healing Arts Institute, Long Beach, CA, 1992

"A Concise Classification of Prescriptions," C.S. Cheung & U. Aik Kaw, *Journal of the Am. Coll. of Traditional Chinese Medicine*, S.F., #4, 1985, pp.14-48

"A Concise Classification of Prescriptions" (continued), C.S. Cheung & U. Aik Kaw, *Journal of the Am. Coll. of Traditional Chinese Medicine*, S.F., # 1-2, 1986, pp. 82-142

Acupuncture: A Comprehensive Text, Shanghai College of Traditional Medicine, translated by Dan Bensky & John O'Connor, Eastland Press, Seattle, 1981

Bi-Syndromes or Rheumatic Disorders Treated by Traditional Chinese Medicine, L. Vangermeersch & Sun Pei-lin, SATAS, Brussels, 1994

Chinese Acupuncture & Moxibustion, Cheng Xinnong, Foreign Languages Press, Beijing, 1987

Chinese-English Terminology of Traditional Chinese Medicine, Shuai Xue-zhong, Hunan Science & Technology Press, Changsha, 1983

Chinese Herbal Medicine: Formulas & Strategies, Dan Bensky & Randall Barolet, Eastland Press, Seattle, 1990

Fluid Physiology & Pathophysiology in Traditional Chinese Medicine, Steven Clavey, Churchill Livingstone, Edinburgh, 1995

Fundamentals of Chinese Medicine, Nigel Wiseman & Andrew Ellis, Paradigm Publications, Brookline, MA, 1985

Glossary of Chinese Medical Terms and Acupuncture Points, Nigel Wiseman, Paradigm Publications, Brookline, MA, 1990

How to Write a TCM Herbal Formula, Bob Flaws, Blue Poppy Press, Boulder, CO, 1993

Principles of Dialectical Differential Diagnosis & Treatment of Traditional Chinese Medicine, C.S. Cheung, Traditional Chinese Medical Publisher, S.F., 1980

Reference Guide to Acupuncture: Zang Fu Principles and Diagnosis, Xie Zhu Fan & William Dunbar, Northern Star Inc., Chicago, 1987

Seventy Essential TCM Herbal Formulas for Beginners, Bob Flaws, Blue Poppy Press, 1994

"Spleen & Stomach Yin Deficiency: Differentiation and Treatment," by Steven Clavey, *Journal of Chinese Medicine*, UK, #47, January 1995

Syndromes of Traditional Chinese Medicine, Huang Bing-shan, Heilongjiang Education Press, Harbin, 1993

The Essentials of Chinese Diagnostics, Manfred Porkert, ACTA Medicinae Sinensis, Chinese Medicine Publications Ltd. Zurich, 1983

The Essential Book of Traditional Chinese Medicine, Vol. 1 & 2, Liu Yanchi, Columbia University Press, NY, 1988

"The Great Qi: Zhang Xichun's Reflections on the Nature, Pathology and Treatment of the *Daqi*," Volker Scheid, *The Journal of Chinese Medicine*, #49, September 1995, pp. 5-16

The Web That Has No Weaver, Ted Kaptchuk, Congdon & Weed, NY, 1983

Traditional Medicine in Contemporary China, Nathan Sivin, Center for Chinese Studies, U. of Michigan, Ann Arbor, 1987

Zang Fu: The Organ System of Traditional Chinese Medicine, Jeremy Ross, Churchill Livingstone, Edinburgh, Second edition, 1988

Formula Index

Symptom Index

A

abdomen, downbearing sensation in the lower 138
abdomen, dull pain in the 69, 70
abdomen, palpable lumps in the upper 148
abdomen, pumping of the legs against the 60
abdomen, sagging and distention in the lower 61
abdomen, severe pain in the lower 30, 117
abdomen, stasis binding in the lower 148
abdominal cold and pain, severe lower 25
abdominal distention and cramping 60
abdominal distention and fatigue after eating 69
abdominal distention and fullness 4, 9, 10, 14, 40, 58, 60, 62, 65, 66, 69, 74-75, 80, 82, 97, 99, 109, 111, 114, 116, 158
abdominal distention, lower 4, 10, 14, 116
abdominal masses when lying supine, visible 147
abdominal pain 29, 33, 54, 55, 62, 64, 70, 107, 121, 148, 149
abdominal pain, enduring lower 149
abdominal pain, lower 29, 54, 55, 121, 148, 149
abdominal pain, mild, persistent 107
abdominal sagging pain, lower 141
abortions, artificial 148
abortion, habitual 61, 62
abscess, intestinal 117
accumulations and gatherings 143
aching, generalized 153
acid eructation 23
acid regurgitation 16, 17, 58, 66, 67, 81
acne 14, 15, 17, 23, 111
acne with swollen, red lesions 111
aging 27, 34-36, 41, 49, 62, 68-70, 104, 105, 110, 115, 120, 123, 126, 128, 176
agitation 14, 42, 46, 47, 49, 51, 79, 89
AIDS 132
alcohol, drinking too much 30, 32, 48, 78, 109, 150
amenorrhea 14, 19, 126, 128, 141, 149
amoebic dysentery 6
anemia 40, 142
anger 9, 10, 12, 14, 15, 21, 22, 32, 42, 45, 47, 78, 101, 138, 146-148, 160, 161
anger, easy 14, 15, 42, 45, 78, 101, 138
anger, intense 21
anger, no constancy in joy and 43
angina pectoris 43
ankle, sprained 3
anus, burning sensation around the 91, 109
anxiety 24, 31, 34, 49, 157

appendicitis, acute 117
appetite, diminished 13, 39, 59, 64, 65 168
asthma 52, 122, 123
auditory acuity, diminished 119

B

back, weakness of the low 119
back pain, lower and upper 156
back stiffness, upper 139
bad breath 58, 59, 66, 78, 79
bao han 30
bedroom taxation 150
befuddled and confused 31
bi, damp, with swelling and pain 170
bi, fixed 171
bi, moving 170
birthing, excessive fatigue during 61
bitter medicinals, erroneous or prolonged use of 59
bleeding 15, 16, 23, 24, 39, 62, 63, 79, 80, 83, 88, 91, 92, 106, 126, 135, 141, 143, 149-151
bleeding due to blood heat 15
bleeding, excessive 149
bleeding gums 79, 80
bleeding of fresh, red blood 91
bleeding, severe 151
bleeding ulcers 83
blindness, night 4, 19, 27, 28
blood clots, dark, purplish, within the phlegm 106
blood heat 15, 150, 151
blood insufficiency 20, 36
blood loss 19, 34-36, 39, 63, 126, 142
blood loss, excessive 39, 63, 126
blood stasis 25, 42, 63, 82, 93, 107, 117, 118, 137, 140, 143-148, 151, 162, 163, 166, 172, 173, 175, 176, 178, 179
blood stasis binding in the epigastrium 147
blood vacuity 4, 10, 12, 13, 18-21, 25, 27, 28, 32, 36-38, 41, 42, 46, 137, 141-145, 163, 164, 176, 178, 179
bodily fatigue 39, 72, 93
bodily heaviness 112, 172, 173
body and limbs, heaviness in the 160
body, cold 24, 69, 105
body, cold feeling in the lower half of the 123
body, wandering pain of the 162
body, fat 160
borborygmus 13, 54, 56, 66, 67, 110

Q

R

OTHER BOOKS ON CHINESE MEDICINE
AVAILABLE FROM BLUE POPPY PRESS

1775 Linden Ave, Boulder, CO 80304
For ordering 1-800-487-9296
PH. 303\447-8372 FAX 303\447-0740

SEVENTY ESSENTIAL TCM FORMULAS FOR BEGINNERS by Bob Flaws, ISBN 0-936185-59-7, $19.95

CHINESE PEDIATRIC MASSAGE THERAPY: A Parent's & Practitioner's Guide to the Prevention & Treatment of Childhood Illness, by Fan Ya-li, ISBN 0-936185-54-6, $12.95

RECENT TCM RESEARCH FROM CHINA, trans. by Charles Chace & Bob Flaws, ISBN 0-936185-56-2, $18.95

EXTRA TREATISES BASED ON INVESTIGATION & INQUIRY: A Translation of Zhu Dan-xi's *Ge Zhi Yu Lun*, by Yang Shou-zhong & Duan Wu-jin, ISBN 0-936185-53-8, $15.95

A NEW AMERICAN ACUPUNCTURE by Mark Seem, ISBN 0-936185-44-9, $21.95

PATH OF PREGNANCY, VOL. I, Gestational Disorders by Bob Flaws, ISBN 0-936185-39-2, $19.95

PATH OF PREGNANCY, Vol. II, A Handbook of Trad. Chin. Postpartum Diseases by Bob Flaws. ISBN 0-936185-42-2, $18.95

HOW TO WRITE A TCM HERBAL FORMULA: A Logical Methodology for the Formulation & Administration of Chinese Herbal Medicine in Decoction, by Bob Flaws, ISBN 0-936185-49-X, $10.95

FULFILLING THE ESSENCE A Handbook of Traditional & Contemporary Treatments for Female Infertility, by Bob Flaws, ISBN 0-936185-48-1, $19.95

Li Dong-yuan's TREATISE ON THE SPLEEN & STOMACH, A Translation of the *Pi Wei Lun* by Yang Shou-zhong & Li Jian-yong, ISBN 0-936185-41-4, $22.95

SCATOLOGY & THE GATE OF LIFE: The Role of the Large Intestine in Immunity by Bob Flaws ISBN 0-936185-20-1 $14.95

MENOPAUSE A Second Spring: Making a Smooth Transition with Traditional Chinese Medicine by Honora Lee Wolfe ISBN 0-936185-18-X $14.95

How to Have A HEALTHY PREGNANCY, HEALTHY BIRTH With Traditional Chinese Medicine by Honora Lee Wolfe, ISBN 0-936185-40-6, $9.95

MIGRAINES & TRADITIONAL CHINESE MEDICINE: A Layperson's Guide by Bob Flaws ISBN 0-936185-15-5 $11.95

STICKING TO THE POINT: A Rational Methodology for the Step by Step Formulation & Administration of an Acupuncture Treatment by Bob Flaws ISBN 0-936185-17-1 $16.95

ENDOMETRIOSIS, INFERTILITY AND TRADITIONAL CHINESE MEDICINE: A Laywoman's Guide by Bob Flaws ISBN 0-936185-14-7 $9.95

THE BREAST CONNECTION: A Lay-woman's Guide to the Treatment of Breast Disease by Chinese Medicine by Honora Lee Wolfe ISBN 0-936185-61-9, $9.95

NINE OUNCES: A Nine Part Program For The Prevention of AIDS in HIV Positive Persons by Bob Flaws ISBN 0-936185-12-0 $9.95

THE TREATMENT OF CANCER BY INTEGRATED CHINESE-WESTERN MEDICINE by Zhang Dai-zhao, trans. by Zhang Ting-liang & Bob Flaws, ISBN 0-936185-11-2, $18.95

A HANDBOOK OF TRADITIONAL CHINESE DERMATOLOGY by Liang Jian-hui, trans. by Zhang Ting-liang & Bob Flaws, ISBN 0-936185-07-4 $15.95

A HANDBOOK OF TRADITIONAL CHINESE GYNECOLOGY by Zhejiang College of TCM, trans. by Zhang Ting-liang, ISBN 0-936185-06-6 (4nd edit.) $22.95

PRINCE WEN HUI'S COOK: Chinese Dietary Therapy by Bob Flaws & Honora Lee Wolfe, ISBN 0-912111-05-4, $12.95 (Published by Paradigm Press, Brookline, MA)

THE DAO OF INCREASING LONGEVITY AND CONSERVING ONE'S LIFE by Anna Lin & Bob Flaws, ISBN 0-936185-24-4 $16.95

FIRE IN THE VALLEY: The TCM Diagnosis and Treatment of Vaginal Diseases by Bob Flaws ISBN 0-936185-25-2 $16.95

HIGHLIGHTS OF ANCIENT ACUPUNCTURE PRESCRIPTIONS trans. by Honora Lee Wolfe & Rose Crescenz ISBN 0-936185-23-6, $14.95

ARISAL OF THE CLEAR: A Simple Guide to Healthy Eating According to Traditional Chinese Medicine by Bob Flaws, ISBN #-936185-27-9 $8.95

PEDIATRIC BRONCHITIS: Its Cause, Diagnosis & Treatment According to Traditional Chinese Medicine trans. by Gao Yu-li and Bob Flaws, ISBN 0-936185-26-0 $15.95

AIDS & ITS TREATMENT ACCORDING TO TRADITIONAL CHINESE MEDICINE by Huang Bing-shan, trans. by Fu-Di & Bob Flaws, ISBN 0-936185-28-7 $24.95

ACUTE ABDOMINAL SYNDROMES: Their Diagnosis & Treatment by Combined Chinese-Western Medicine by Alon Marcus, ISBN 0-936185-31-7 $16.95

MY SISTER, THE MOON: The Diagnosis & Treatment of Menstrual Diseases by Traditional Chinese Medicine by Bob Flaws, ISBN 0-936185-34-1, $24.95

FU QING-ZHU'S GYNECOLOGY trans. by Yang Shou-zhong and Liu Da-wei, ISBN 0-936185-35-X, $22.95

FLESHING OUT THE BONES: The Importance of Case Histories in Chinese Medicine trans. by Charles Chace. ISBN 0-936185-30-9, $18.95

CLASSICAL MOXIBUSTION SKILLS in Contemporary Clinical Practice by Sung Baek, ISBN 0-936185-16-3 $12.95

THE MEDICAL I CHING: Oracle of the Healer Within by Miki Shima, OMD, ISBN 0-936185-38-4, $19.95

MASTER TONG'S ACUPUNCTURE: An Ancient Lineage for Modern Practice, trans. and commentary by Miriam Lee, OMD, ISBN 0-936185-37-6, $19.95

A HANDBOOK OF TCM UROLOGY & MALE SEXUAL DYSFUNCTION by Anna Lin, OMD, ISBN 0-936185-36-8, $16.95

PMS: Its Cause, Diagnosis & Treatment According to Traditional Chinese Medicine by Bob Flaws ISBN 0-936185-22-8 $14.95

MASTER HUA'S CLASSIC OF THE CENTRAL VISCERA by Hua Tuo, ISBN 0-936185-43-0, $21.95

THE HEART & ESSENCE OF DAN-XI'S METHODS OF TREATMENT by Xu Dan-xi, trans. by Yang Shou-zhong, ISBN 0-926185-49-X, $21.95

STATEMENTS OF FACT IN TRADITIONAL CHINESE MEDICINE by Bob Flaws, ISBN 0-936185-52-X, $12.95

IMPERIAL SECRETS OF HEALTH & LONGEVITY by Bob Flaws, ISBN 0-936185-51-1, $9.95

THE SYSTEMATIC CLASSIC OF ACUPUNCTURE & MOXIBUSTION (*Jia Yi Jing*) by Huang-fu Mi, trans. by Yang Shou-zhong and Charles Chace, ISBN 0-936185-29-5, $79.95

CHINESE MEDICINAL WINES & ELIXIRS by Bob Flaws, ISBN 0-936185-58-9, $18.95

THE DIVINELY RESPONDING CLASSIC:
A Translation of the *Shen Ying Jing* from *Zhen Jiu Da Cheng*, trans. by Yang Shou-zhong & Liu Feng-ting ISBN 0-936185-55-4, $15.95

PAO ZHI: An Introduction to Processing Chinese Medicinals to Enhance Their Therapeutic Effect, by Philippe Sionneau, ISBN 0-936185-62-1, $34.95

THE BOOK OF JOOK: Chinese Medicinal Porridges, An Alternative to the Typical Western Breakfast, by Bob Flaws, ISBN0-936185-60-0, $16.95

SHAOLIN SECRET FORMULAS for the Treatment of External Injuries, by De Chan, ISBN 0-936185-08-2, $18.95

AGING & BLOOD STASIS: A New Approach to TCM Geriatrics, by Yan De-xin, ISBN 0-936185-63-5, $21.95

CHINESE MEDICAL PALMISTRY: Your Health in Your Hand, by Zong Xiao-fan & Gary Liscum, ISBN 0-936185-64-3, $15.95

THE SECRET OF CHINESE PULSE DIAGNOSIS by Bob Flaws, ISBN 0-936185-67-8, $17.95

LOW BACK PAIN: Care & Prevention with Traditional Chinese Medicine by Douglas Frank, ISBN 0-936185-66-X, $9.95

THE TREATMENT OF DISEASE IN TCM:
Vol. I, Diseases of the Head and Face by Philippe Sionneau, ISBN 0-936185-69-4, $21.95

ACUPUNCTURE AND MOXIBUSTION FORMULAS & TREATMENTS by Cheng Dan-an, trans. By Wu Ming, ISBN 0-936185-68-6, $22.95